Clinics in Developmental Medicine No. 128
THE MANAGEMENT OF VISUAL IMPAIRMENT IN CHILDHOOD

Clinics in Developmental Medicine No. 128

The Management of Visual Impairment in Childhood

Edited by: ALISTAIR R. FIELDER
University of Birmingham Medical School

ANTHONY B. BEST
University of Birmingham

MARTIN C. O. BAX
Community Paediatric Research Unit
Chelsea and Westminster Hospital

1993
Mac Keith Press

Distributed by 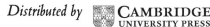 CAMBRIDGE
UNIVERSITY PRESS

©1993 Mac Keith Press
5a Netherhall Gardens, London NW3 5RN

First published in this edition 1993

British Library Cataloguing-in-Publication data:
A catalogue record for this book is available from the British Library

ISSN 0069-4835

0 521 451507

Printed in Great Britain at The Lavenham Press Ltd., Lavenham, Suffolk
Mac Keith Press is supported by **The Spastics Society, London, England**

CONTENTS

CONTRIBUTORS

STUART AITKEN, BSc, PhD — Research Fellow, Communication Aids for Language and Learning, University of Edinburgh

JANETTE ATKINSON, PhD — MRC Senior Scientist, Visual Development Unit, University of Cambridge

GILLIAN BAIRD, FRCP — Consultant Developmental Paediatrician, Guy's Hospital, London

MARTIN C.O. BAX, DM, FRCP — Senior Research Fellow, Community Paediatric Research Unit, Chelsea and Westminster Hospital, London

JUDY BELL — Headteacher, RNIB Sunshine House School, Southport, Lancashire

ANTHONY B. BEST, MEd, DipEd(VH), DipAES(Deaf) — Headteacher, RNIB Condover Hall School, Shrewsbury; Lecturer in Special Education, University of Birmingham

MARIANNA BUULTJENS, MA, DipCTB — Senior Lecturer, Moray House Institute, Edinburgh

JANET EDWARDS — Director and Joint Principal, Woodcroft School, Loughton, Essex

ALISTAIR R. FIELDER, MRCP, FRCS, FCOphth — Professor of Ophthalmology, Department of Ophthalmology, University of Birmingham Medical School, Birmingham

CLARE GILBERT, MB, ChB, FRCS, FCOphth — Research Fellow, Department of Preventive Ophthalmology, Institute of Ophthalmology, University of London

WILLIAM V. GOOD, MD — Assistant Professor, Department of Ophthalmology, University of California, USA

ROBERT GREENHALGH, BA, CSW — Principal of Training, South Regional Association for the Blind, London

MARYKE GROENVELD, PhD, RPsych — Visually Impaired Program, Department of Pediatrics, British Columbia's Children's Hospital, Vancouver, BC, Canada

JAMES E. JAN, MD, FRCP(C) — Professor, Visually Impaired Program, Department of Pediatrics, British Columbia's Children's Hospital, Vancouver, BC, Canada

ANTHONY T. MOORE, MA, FRCS, FCOphth — Consultant Ophthalmic Surgeon, Addenbrooke's Hospital, Cambridge; *and* Moorfields Eye Hospital, London

JACQUELINE NICHOLSON — Consultant Community Paediatrician (Special Needs), Community Health Services, NHS Trust, Southern Derbyshire

PATRICIA M. SONKSEN, MD, MRCP — Senior Lecturer in Developmental Paediatrics, The Wolfson Centre, Neurosciences Unit, Institute of Child Health, London

MICHAEL J. TOBIN — Director, Research Centre for the Education of the Visually Handicapped, School of Education, University of Birmingham

JACKIE VAN HOF-VAN DUIN, MD, PhD — Associate Professor of Physiology, Department of Physiology I, Erasmus University, Rotterdam, The Netherlands

PREFACE

In most developed countries the prevalence of significant visual impairment among children aged under 15 is well below 1:1000, so that for most practitioners working in child health (even ophthalmologists) experience of these children will not be extensive. Yet in the course of practice every clinician will at some time be confronted with a child with a permanent visual problem. This creates a dilemma, as the clinician may well not have the relevant experience to understand the intricacies of this complex situation, and the child and family thus may not always receive the appropriate care and advice. The problem is amplified as nearly two-thirds of visually impaired children have other difficulties as well. Clearly training is the answer, though few areas have recognized centres of training. Hopefully this book can help fill that gap. Just as it is not easy for the clinician to gain the relevant experience, so the editors of this book knew that to obtain a reasonably comprehensive account of visual disability in childhood would be difficult and that an international effort would be required. We are grateful, therefore, to authors on both sides of the Atlantic for their contributions.

When it came to writing about the provision of services at a local level, inevitably it was necessary to draw on individual experience gained at the relevant centres. This means that some chapters make reference to local situations which are specific to the country in which the author resides. However, the principles of management are the same throughout the world.

While we are pleased with the comprehensive accounts of most aspects of the diagnosis, treatment and management of the visually disabled child, we know that we have not included a chapter that we dearly wanted to, concerning the adolescent and young adult with a visual disability, and the problems of entering the work place and/or finding a suitable vocation in adult life. As in other aspects of disability (see Thomas *et al.* 1989), the development of services for adolescents and young adults is patchy and we knew of no-one with sufficient experience in the field to give us clear guidance about how services should be developed. We hope this lacuna is one that some of our readers will fill in the future.

As the book came together the paucity of information and literature on many important topics became glaringly apparent. For instance, the past decade has seen an explosion of interest in visual development, with the introduction of exciting, clinically relevant methods of evaluating visual function in infancy and early childhood. To date, however, their impact on children with low vision is minimal. This is due not to test inadequacy but rather to a failure of clinicians and scientists to see the challenge. This is changing, but at present we still do not really understand functional vision—such a fundamental issue for education and everyday living.

The visually disabled child, even when there are no additional disabilities, presents one of the greatest challenges to the health and educational professions in meeting the child's needs. The emphasis of this book is on health needs, but we also present accounts of the educational and social implications of visual impairment. We hope that the health professional will thus be able to comprehend what colleagues in the social services and in education are attempting to do to help the child. Contributors offer insight into current educational issues and technological innovations. Although of course many of the latter will rapidly be superceded, the point is that management of the visually disabled child is team work and requires input from a range of professions, with whom the clinician must be in contact.

Perhaps one other deficiency of this book is the lack of a contribution by a visually disabled young person, but throughout (for example in the chapter by Maryke Groenveld) there are vignettes of the problems that young people with this disability have encountered. Also included are ideas on how to help and solve these problems. The aim of this book is to ensure that the visually disabled child receives the very best service possible.

ALISTAIR R. FIELDER
ANTHONY B. BEST
MARTIN C.O. BAX

REFERENCE

Thomas, A.P., Bax, M.C.O., Smyth, D.P.L. (1989) *The Health and Social Needs of Young Adults with Physical Disabilities. Clinics in Developmental Medicine No. 106.* London: Mac Keith Press.

1
EPIDEMIOLOGY

Gillian Baird and Anthony T. Moore

There are thought to be more than one million blind children in the world and a greater number with lesser but significant degrees of visual impairment (VI) (Foster 1988). Much of this visually disabling disease is preventable, but before any initiatives for prevention and treatment can be planned or undertaken, there needs to be clear information about the prevalence of childhood VI and the major causes. Although there are a large number of different publications on this subject, most studies have serious limitations, and because of the different definitions of VI, the different age groups and populations studied and different methods of presenting the data it is difficult to correlate the information from these sources. There has been no consistent definition of either childhood or blindness. Most studies suffer from low ascertainment and, since information has usually been collected from blind schools or blind registration statistics, there has been under-reporting of multiply disabled children whose VI forms part of a more widespread neuro-developmental disorder. Community based studies (Bryars and Archer 1977, Goggin and O'Keefe 1991) suggest that 40 to 50 per cent of blind children have other disabilities, and it is important that these children are included in any assessment of the problem. In this review we will attempt to make an assessment of the prevalence and major causes of childhood VI in different areas of the world and briefly consider how some of these disorders may be prevented.

Definition
One of the major problems in assessing the prevalence of childhood VI in different studies is the large number of different definitions that have been used (Cullinan 1987). It would be helpful if agreement could be reached to use a common definition of childhood, perhaps the UNICEF range of birth to 15 years. The World Health Organization (1980) has published definitions of normal vision and of varying degrees of VI (Table 1.1). Although visual acuity is the most widely used measure of visual function, the WHO definitions also cover other aspects of visual function such as nyctalopia, visual field loss and diplopia. These definitions are of limited value in studies of childhood VI because of the difficulty in quantifying visual acuity in young infants, and in older children with mental retardation, without the use of sophisticated techniques. Gilbert *et al.* (1993) have recently designed a standardized form for collecting data on childhood VI which if generally accepted and used will allow valid comparisons to be made between different studies. However, other problems such as standardization of testing conditions

1

TABLE 1.1
WHO terminology for visual impairment*

Category of vision	Degree of impairment	Best corrected visual acuity	Alternative definition
Normal vision	None	≥0.8 (6/7.5)	—
	Slight	<0.8	Near-normal
Low vision	Moderate	<0.3 (6/18)	Moderate low vision
	Severe	<0.12 (6/48)	Severe low vision. Counting fingers at 6m or less
Blindness	Profound	<0.05 (3/60)	Profound low vision or moderate blindness. Counting fingers at <3m
	Near-total	<0.02 (1/60)	Severe or near total blindness. Counting fingers at 1m or less or hand movements at 5m or less
	Total	No light perception (NPL)	Total blindness (including absence of the eye)

*World Health Organization (1980).

(Cullinan 1987), coding of diseases, and the recording of causes of restricted vision in each eye (especially when they differ) remain and need to be resolved (Johnson and Minassian 1989).

Prevalence

Although most studies of childhood VI suffer from low ascertainment and may have sources of bias, it is possible to obtain some approximate figures of prevalence. It is evident from published studies that there is great variation in the prevalence in different parts of the world. Bryars and Archer (1977) in a community based study in Northern Ireland found a prevalence of VI (defined as a visual acuity of 6/18 or less in the better eye) of 81/100,000. Most children were examined by the same ophthalmologist and ascertainment was estimated at 80 per cent. Blindness registration statistics from England and Wales (using a definition of blindness of 3/60 or less in the better eye) give a prevalence of about 32/100,000 in childhood (Cullinan 1987), which is in agreement with figures calculated by Robinson et al. (1987) in Canada and Riise et al. (1992) in Scandinavia using similar sources and definition. Blindness registration statistics, however, may seriously underestimate the prevalence of childhood VI (Bruce et al. 1991, Evans and Wormold 1993), and in England and Wales where the Department for Education also collects statistics of children with VI derived from school returns there is a clear discrepancy between these figures and those derived from registration statistics and government surveys of disability (Fine 1979, Walker et al. 1992). Goggins and O'Keefe (1992) in their community based study in the Republic of Ireland found that 108 out of a total of 172 blind children were unregistered. A

TABLE 1.2

Visual impairment in children in West Sussex*

Total population 0–15 years	152,000
Total visually impaired	99
Blind (vision 3/60 or worse)	18
Blind one eye, low vision (6/24–6/60) other eye	24
Low vision both eyes	57
Multiple disabilities	60
Cerebral palsy or severe motor deficit	31
Epilepsy	12
Deafness	9
Additional structural malformation	10

*Data compiled from special needs register and validated by Dr Ann Abra, Consultant Community Paediatrician.

    Of the 99 visually impaired children, 46 were unable to perform formal tests of visual acuity. An ocular diagnosis was recorded in 73 children, and 20 had evidence of visual pathway damage.

recent survey in the UK by the Royal National Institute for the Blind (Bruce *et al.* 1991) estimated that blindness and partial sight are under-registered by 64 per cent and 77 per cent respectively in the adult population, and it is likely that the situation is as bad in respect of childhood VI, especially amongst children with multiple disabilities (Walker *et al.* 1992). Many health authorities in the UK are now seeking to keep registers of children with special needs, and these may give more accurate assessments of the prevalence of childhood VI. It is however important to validate the register at frequent intervals (Colver 1989). One such register is that of West Sussex which was validated in 1990 (Table 1.2). The prevalence of low vision (defined as 6/24 or less) in this child population is 65 per 100,000 (26/100,000 have no other disabling condition and 12/100,000 have vision of 3/60 or less in the better eye).

    In contrast, a random population based study in Malawi using the WHO definition of blindness found a prevalence of 110/100,000 in children under 6 years of age (Chirambo *et al.* 1986). Although these figures reflect only information in early childhood, it is evident that the prevalence of blindness in Africa, for example, is many times greater than that seen in the UK and North America. Similarly high prevalence rates are reported for Asia and South America (Cohen *et al.* 1985, Gilbert *et al.* 1993). The true extent of the blinding diseases is even greater, as infants with acquired VI from measles and vitamin A deficiency have an extremely high mortality rate. Moreover, the major causes in the developing world are quite different from those in the industrialized nations.

Aetiology

There is unfortunately no generally agreed format for recording the causes of visual loss in children, and the methods used in different studies have varied. Some have

TABLE 1.3
Aetiology of visual impairment in published studies

Study	Country	N	Setting	Major causes
Fraser and Friedman (1967)	UK	776	Blind schools	Genetic (42%) Perinatal (33%)
Olurin (1970)	Nigeria	140	Hospital clinic	Acquired disease*
Hatfield (1972)	US	3115	State agencies	Genetic (47%)
Linstedt (1972)	Sweden	515	Blind schools	Pre- and perinatal causes (90%) Postnatal causes (10%)
Merin et al. (1972)	Cyprus	112	Blind schools	Genetic (80%)
Baghdassarian and Tabbara (1975)	Lebanon	230	Blind schools	Genetic (77%)
Chirambo and Benezra (1976)	Malawi	270	Blind school	Infection (75%—measles 44%)
Bryars and Archer (1977)	Northern Ireland	486	Community	Genetic (51%) Perinatal (21%)
Tabbara and Badr (1985)	Saudi Arabia	187	Blind school	Genetic (84%)
Van der Pol (1986)	Holland	1334	Blind schools	Genetic (46%)
Robinson et al. (1987)	Canada	576	Blind register	Genetic*
Rosenberg (1987)	Denmark	150	Blind register	Genetic (29%) Perinatal (23%)
Phillips et al. (1987)	Scotland	99	Blind school	Genetic (48%)
Moriarty (1988)	Jamaica	108	Blind schools	Genetic (48%) Congenital rubella (22%)
Rojas et al. (1990)	Peru	202	Blind school	Acquired disease (47%) Infections (21%)
Goggin and O'Keefe (1991)	Eire	172	Community	Perinatal (27%) Genetic (18%)
Gilbert et al. (1993)	W. Africa	284	Blind school	Acquired disease (30%) Genetic (20%)
	S. India	305	Blind school	Acquired disease (33%) Genetic (30%)
	Chile	217	Blind school	Genetic (30%) Perinatal (20%)

*Detailed breakdowns not available.

used an anatomical classification, while in other studies an attempt has been made to assess the aetiology of the blinding disease. We believe that both approaches are useful, but the aetiological classification helps highlight the areas in which disease prevention may be effective and we have therefore tried to assess the various reports in this way (Table 1.3). (An analysis of the anatomical causes of blindness is given in Chapter 16.) It is helpful to consider whether the disorders are *genetically determined* or caused by *intrauterine events* (*e.g.* rubella), *perinatal factors* (*e.g.* retinopathy of prematurity or perinatal hypoxia) or *acquired disease* (*e.g.* corneal infections).

Developing countries
Information about the causes of childhood VI in developing countries comes almost

exclusively from blind school surveys and assessment of children seen in hospital eye clinics. Although these children may not be representative of the broad population of children with VI, such studies may give useful information about the major causes of VI in childhood. For example, the community based study from Malawi (Chirambo *et al.* 1986) showed good agreement in the causes of childhood blindness with a previous blind school survey (Chirambo and Benezra 1976) in the same country.

Bilateral corneal scarring, acquired in early childhood, is responsible for over half the cases of childhood VI in Africa (Chirambo and Benezra 1976, Sandford-Smith and Whittle 1979, Chirambo *et al.* 1986, Foster 1988) but for less than 1 per cent of those in Europe and North America (Fraser and Friedmann 1967, Hatfield 1972, Bryars and Archer 1977). Several different but interrelated factors, including malnutrition, vitamin A deficiency, measles and herpes simplex virus infections, and the use of traditional eye medicine, are involved in the aetiology of the keratitis and subsequent corneal scarring. The mechanism of the corneal scarring has been reviewed in detail by Foster (1988). Other major causes in Africa include ophthalmia neonatorum, cataract, congenital glaucoma and uveitis (Olurin 1970, Chirambo and Benezra 1976, Foster 1988). Most of this blindness occurs in otherwise normal children. Genetic diseases are responsible for less than 10 per cent of cases of childhood blindness (Chirambo and Benezra 1976). Retinopathy of prematurity (ROP) and visual pathway damage are similarly rare causes of VI. This reflects the enormous differences in paediatric care and childhood mortality rates between Europe and North America and developing countries. In Africa, for example, preterm infants and those with perinatal hypoxia or complex genetic disorders rarely survive and are therefore not seen in blind schools or hospital clinics.

Acquired, particularly corneal, disease is similarly the leading cause of childhood VI in deprived communities in Asia and South America (Rojas *et al.* 1990, Gilbert *et al.* 1993). However, in countries such as Chile where there is effective measles vaccination and where vitamin A deficiency is not a major health problem, ROP and genetic diseases are more common (Gilbert *et al.* 1993). In the Caribbean, where there is less malnutrition and better medical services, congenital rubella is the leading preventable cause of VI, accounting for 22 per cent of children in blind schools in one study in Jamaica (Moriarty 1988). Overall, genetic disease accounted for 48 per cent of cases of childhood blindness. Similar studies in Saudi Arabia (Tabbara and Badr 1985), Cyprus (Merin *et al.* 1972) and the Lebanon (Baghdassarian and Tabbara 1975) have shown that genetic diseases account for about 80 per cent of cases of childhood blindness. This high figure, due predominantly to autosomal recessive disease, is related to the high proportion of consanguineous marriages in these communities.

Europe and North America
Most of the information about causes of childhood VI in Europe has come either

5

from surveys of blind schools (Fraser and Friedmann 1967, Lindstedt 1972, Van der Pol 1986, Phillips *et al.* 1987) or from blindness registration statistics (Fine 1979, Cullinan 1987, Riise *et al.* 1992, Rosenberg *et al.* 1992). Both of these sources are biased toward the reporting of otherwise normal blind children and may underestimate the contribution of visual pathway damage which is more common in the multiply disabled child (Warburg *et al.* 1979). Only two community based studies have been published (Bryars and Archer 1977, Goggin and O'Keefe 1992).

It is evident both from those community based studies and from studies from blind schools (Fraser and Friedmann 1967, Lindstedt 1972, Van der Pol 1986, Phillips *et al.* 1987) and blindness registers (Riise *et al.* 1992, Rosenberg *et al.* 1992) that genetic disease is the single most important aetiological factor, accounting for between 40 and 50 per cent of all childhood blindness. In contrast to studies from the Middle East (Merin *et al.* 1972, Baghdassarian and Tabbara 1975, Tabbara and Badr 1985), where genetic disease is also common, autosomal dominant disease is at least as common as recessive disorders, X-linked disorders accounting for less than 10 per cent of all genetic disease. Congenital cataract, inherited retinal dystrophies and albinism are the most common genetic disorders (Fraser and Friedmann 1967, Bryars and Archer 1977, Phillips *et al.* 1987, Goggin and O'Keefe 1992, Riise *et al.* 1992, Rosenberg *et al.* 1992). Non-genetic congenital malformations, predominantly congenital glaucoma and microphthalmos, account for about 8 per cent of blind children (Fraser and Friedmann 1967, Bryars and Archer 1977).

The second most important cause of VI is perinatal disease, predominantly visual pathway damage associated with birth hypoxia and ROP. In the study by Fraser and Friedmann (1967), ROP was aetiological in 177 (23 per cent) of 760 children with VI surveyed. These children were born in the 1950s when there was a much higher incidence of ROP than today. Severe cicatricial ROP has become a disease of much smaller infants, predominantly those <1000g, many of whom have additional neurological impairments (Robinson *et al.* 1987, Hoon *et al.* 1988). Although in the more recent study of Bryars and Archer (1977) ROP still accounted for 12 per cent of cases of childhood blindness, a more important cause was visual pathway disease which accounted for 42 per cent of cases. It is uncommon for CNS damage to be confined to the visual pathway, and most of these children have additional neurological impairment. Congenital cataract remains the most important diagnosis among children who are partially sighted (Bryars and Archer 1977), and there is some evidence that advances in the management of this disorder have moved this group of children from the category of 'blind' to that of 'partially sighted' (Robinson *et al.* 1987). In contrast to the situation in the developing world, disease acquired in later childhood due to infection, trauma or tumours is an uncommon cause of childhood blindness in Europe. Studies from North America (Hatfield 1972, Robinson *et al.* 1987) show a similar picture. In the 1950s cicatricial ROP was the leading cause of childhood VI but more recently the numbers have declined (Hoon *et al.* 1988). There has been a similar decline in the importance of congenital rubella as a cause of visual morbidity. The two major aetiological factors are now genetic disease and perinatal hypoxia, and the most common disorders causing VI are congenital cataract, inherited retinal dystrophies and optic atrophy or other visual pathway damage (Lindstedt 1972, Bryars and Archer 1977, Van der Pol 1986). The majority of blind children now have additional impairments, mostly neurodevelopmental disorders (Bryars and Archer 1977, Van der Pol 1986).

Prevention

In Africa and deprived areas of Asia and South America, much of the childhood VI is, theoretically at least, preventable with simple and inexpensive measures. Widespread provision of dietary advice, vitamin A supplementation and fortification of staple foods, topical antibiotics and measles vaccination would have a major effect in reducing the incidence of blinding disease (Foster 1988). However, there remain formidable logistic, financial and political difficulties in introducing effective programmes for preventing VI. In many countries the high prevalence of childhood VI is an indicator of general economic difficulties, and where the overall health budget is small and where there are other major health problems, the prevention of VI may not be a high priority.

In other areas of the developing world such as the Caribbean and South America where health care services are more advanced, the introduction of rubella vaccination would have a significant effect on the incidence of childhood VI. In the more prosperous societies of Europe and North America, most severe childhood VI is due to genetic disease or to visual pathway damage associated with perinatal hypoxia. Early diagnosis and treatment may improve the prognosis in some infants, for example those with ROP, congenital cataract and congenital glaucoma, but in most cases there is no effective treatment. The prevention of blindness from genetic disease and perinatal problems represents a major challenge for the next decade. The subject is discussed at length in Chapter 16.

REFERENCES

Baghdassarian, S.A., Tabbara, K.F. (1975) 'Childhood blindness in Lebanon.' *American Journal of Ophthalmology*, **79**, 827–830.

Bruce, L, McKennell, A., Walker, A.E. (1991) *Blind and Partially Sighted Adults in Britain: the RNIB Survey*. London: HMSO.

Bryars, J.H., Archer, D.B. (1977) 'Aetiological survey of visually handicapped children in Northern Ireland.' *Transactions of the Ophthalmological Society of the United Kingdom*, **97**, 26–29.

Chirambo, M.C., Benezra, D. (1976) 'Causes of blindness among students in blind school institutions in a developing country.' *British Journal of Ophthalmology*, **60**, 665–668.

—— Tielsch, J.M., West, K.P., Katz, J., Tizazu, T., Schwab, L., Johnson, G., Swartwood, J., Taylor, H.R., Sommer, A. (1986) 'Blindness and visual impairment in Southern Malawi.' *Bulletin of the World Health Organization*, **64**, 567–572.

Cohen, N., Rahman, H., Sprague, J., Jahl, M., Limbuis, E., Mitra, M. (1985) 'Prevalence and determinants of nutritional blindness in Bangladeshi children.' *World Health Statistical Quarterly*, **38**, 317–329.

Colver, A.F., Robinson, A. (1989) 'Establishing a register of children with special needs.' *Archives of Disease in Childhood*, **64**, 1200–1203.

Cullinan, T.R. (1987) 'The epidemiology of blindness.' *In:* Miller, S. (Ed.) *Clinical Ophthalmology.* London: Wright, pp. 571–578.

Evans, J.R., Wormold, R.P.L. (1993) 'Epidemiological function of the BD8 certification.' *Eye*, **7**, 172–179.

Fine, S.R. (1979) 'Incidence of visual handicap in childhood.' *In:* Smith, V., Keen, J. (Eds) *Visual Handicap in Childhood. Clinics in Developmental Medicine No. 73.* London: Spastics International Medical Publications, pp. 36–41.

Foster, A. (1988) 'Childhood blindness.' *Eye*, Suppl 2, 13–18.

Fraser, G., Friedmann, A.I. (1967) *The Causes of Blindness in Childhood.* Baltimore: Johns Hopkins University Press.

Gilbert, G.E., Canovas, R., Hagan, M., Rao, S., Foster, A. (1993) 'Causes of childhood blindness: results from West Africa, South India and Chile.' *Eye*, **7**, 184–188.

Goggin, M., O'Keefe, M. (1991) 'Childhood blindness in the Republic of Ireland.' *British Journal of Ophthalmology*, **75**, 425–429.

Hatfield, E.M. (1972) 'Blindness in infants and young children.' *Sight Saving Review*, **42**, 69–89.

Hoon, A.H., Jan, J.E., Whitfield, M.F., McCormick, A.Q., Richards, C.P., Robinson, G.C. (1988) 'Changing pattern of retinopathy of prematurity: a 37 year clinic experience.' *Pediatrics*, **82**, 344—348.

Johnson, G.J., Minassian, D.C. (1989) 'Prevalence of blindness and eye disease: discussion paper.' *Journal of the Royal Society of Medicine*, **82**, 351-354.

Lindstdt, E. (1972) 'Severe visual impairment in Swedish schoolchildren.' *Documenta Ophthalmologica*, **31**, 172–204.

Merin, S., Lapithis, A.G., Horovitz, D., Michaelson, I.C. (1972) 'Childhood blindness in Cyprus.' *American Journal of Ophthalmology*, **74**, 539–542.

Moriarty, B. (1988) 'Childhood blindness in Jamaica.' *British Journal of Ophthalmology*, **72**, 65–67.

Olurin, O. (1970) 'Etiology of blindness in Nigerian children.' *American Journal of Ophthalmology*, **70**, 533–539.

Phillips, C.I., Levy, A.M., Newton, M., Stokoe, L.N. (1987) 'Blindness in schoolchildren: importance of hereditary, congenital cataract and prematurity.' *British Journal of Ophthalmology*, **71**, 578–584.

Riise, R., Flage, T., Hansen, E., Rosenberg, T., Rudanko, S-L., Viggosson, G., Warburg, M. (1992) 'Visual impairment in Nordic children. I. Nordic registers and prevalence data.' *Acta Ophthalmologica*, **70**, 145–154.

Robinson, G.C., Jan, J.E., Kinnis, C. (1987) 'Congenital ocular blindness in children, 1945–1984.' *American Journal of Diseases of Children*, **145**, 1321–1324.

Rojas, J.R., Lavado, L., Echegaray, L. (1990) 'Childhood blindness in Peru.' *Annals of Ophthalmology*, **22**, 423–425.

Rosenberg, T. (1987) 'Visual impairment in Danish children 1985.' *Acta Ophthalmologica*, **65**, 110—117.

—— Flage, T., Hansen, E., Rudanko, S-L., Viggosson, G., Riise, R. (1992) 'Visual impairment in Nordic children. II. Aetiological factors.' *Acta Olphthalmologica*, **70**, 155–164.

Sandford-Smith, J.H., Whittle, H.C. (1979) 'Corneal ulceration following measles in Nigerian children.' *British Journal of Ophthalmology*, **63**, 720–724.

Tabbara, K.F., Badr, I.A. (1985) 'Changing pattern of childhood blindness in Saudi Arabia.' *British Journal of Ophthalmology*, **69**, 312–315.

Van der Pol, B.A.E. (1986) 'Causes of visual impairment in children.' *Documenta Ophthalmologica*, **61**, 223–228.

Walker, E., Tobin, M., McKennel, A. (1992) *Blind and Partially Sighted Children in Britain: the RNIB Survey.* London: HMSO.

Warburg, M., Frederiksen, P., Ratleff, J. (1979) 'Blindness among 7700 mentally retarded children in Denmark.' *In:* Smith, V., Keen, J. (Eds) *Visual Handicap in Children. Clinics in Developmental Medicine No. 73.* London: Spastics International Medical Publications, pp. 56–67.

World Health Organization (1980) *International Classification of Impairments, Disabilities, and Handicaps.* Geneva: WHO.

2
VISUAL ASSESSMENT DURING THE FIRST YEARS OF LIFE

Janette Atkinson and Jackie Van Hof-van Duin

In recent years, clinical methods have been devised which allow the quantitative assessment of behavioural and electrophysiological visual function in infants and young children. These methods require no verbal capacity or motor skills on the part of the child. They have allowed researchers to gauge the time course of normal development for discrimination of various visual attributes such as colour, shape and depth and to study the development of visual attentional mechanisms. They have also proved very useful in diagnosing and assessing abnormal visual development.

This chapter presents a brief overview of paediatric visual defects and a summary of assessment methods used by two different teams, one in the Netherlands and one in the UK. Not all the techniques described are exclusive to these two centres. Whenever possible, data on both normal and abnormal development are reported. The final section summarizes some of the questions to be answered by liaison between basic and clinical research in the future.

Paediatric visual problems
These vary widely in their severity, and can be divided into two groups comprising (1) those involving mild or no visual disability (*e.g.* strabismus, amblyopia, refractive errors), and (2) those causing a severe disabling impairment ranging from partial sight to complete blindness (*e.g.* cataracts, glaucoma retinoblastoma and cortical blindness).

Children in developed countries with severe visual impairment are fortunately rare (although estimates of prevalence vary widely between 2/10,000 and 3/1000 depending on definition), whereas mild visual impairments are very common (prevalence of strabismus, amblyopia and significant refractive error in preschool children is estimated at 2 to 10 per cent depending on population and definition). It has been estimated that 20,000 children born each year within the UK will become strabismic in the preschool years, with most becoming so in the first two years of life (Medical Research Council 1989).

The extent of disability resulting from the common visual defects of strabismus (commonly called 'squint') and amblyopia is controversial. For example, many people have noted that strabismus carries with it a whole range of possible consequences (many unmeasured and unquantifiable), from difficulties with social

9

interactions and communication, to visuomotor problems affecting tasks such as walking upstairs. Others have considered strabismus in isolation a defect but not a disability (SPORU 1991). This controversy runs throughout the paediatric vision literature and stems from lack of detailed research on paediatric visual disability. The concept of visual disability has not been clearly defined in an age-specific way for infants and children and we therefore lack clear guidelines for definitions of partial sight and blindness. We also lack knowledge about the interdependency between visual development and motor, cognitive and social development, and whether developmental problems in different domains are correlated or causally linked in individual children.

In addition, recent studies of dyslexia have suggested that visual defects (*e.g.* poor control of convergence, abnormal eye movements, defects of the transient visual system) can play a significant role in the syndrome. While many would be unhappy calling 'dyslexia' a visual defect, it is obviously a prevalent paediatric disability which can be associated with certain visual disorders where there may be visual precursors in infancy. Visual dyslexia can be considered a severe disability in educational terms, but a mild one in terms of everyday functional vision.

Paediatric visual problems can also be divided into: (1) those with a visual defect in isolation (*i.e.* with largely normal motor, cognitive and social development), and (2) those with more than one major defect including vision (*i.e.* multiple disabilities), of which the largest group consists of those with cerebral palsy.

In a recent report in the UK by the Royal National Institute for the Blind (1990), the second group has been called multihandicapped visually impaired (MHVI). It has been estimated that there are around 21,000 visually impaired individuals aged 0–19 years in the UK, and at a conservative estimate around 6000 of these would be classified as MHVI. The latter figure is likely to be an underestimate due to the difficulties with both assessment and diagnosis of children under 2 years.

Given these estimates of paediatric visual defects, what attempts can be made to assess abnormality by comparison with normative data concerning various aspects of vision? The approaches of two different groups to this question are considered below.

Visual assessment in Rotterdam, The Netherlands
The present studies in the Department of Physiology I, Erasmus University, Rotterdam, address the question of which groups of children are at risk for abnormal visual development (whether only delayed, or permanently impaired) and at which age visual defects can be demonstrated.

In this laboratory, visual development is studied by examining four functions: visual acuity, visual fields, optokinetic nystagmus and the visual threat response.

Visual acuity
Visual acuity is assessed by means of the preferential looking technique (Teller *et*

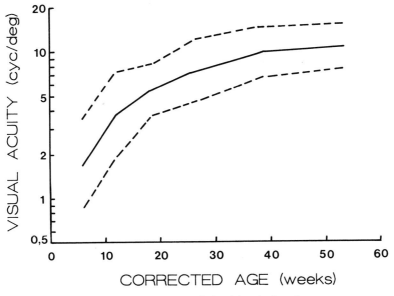

Fig. 2.1. Development of visual (grating) acuity.

al. 1974, Dobson and Teller 1978, Van Hof-van Duin and Mohn 1986*a*) or the acuity card procedure (MacDonald *et al.* 1975, Mohn *et al.* 1988). These methods are based on the inborn preference for a pattern as opposed to a uniform comparison field. The child sits or is held in front of a uniform grey screen. On one side of the screen there is a black and white pattern and on the other side there is a 'blank' (which in fact consists of a very fine pattern assumed to be unresolvable by the infant). An observer watches the infant's face from behind the screen through a peephole located between the stimulus positions. Gratings of different stripe widths are presented with the left–right position of the pattern varied randomly from trial to trial. The observer, who is unaware of the left–right position of the grating stimulus, is required to judge the stimulus position on the basis of the infant's eye and head movements. Starting with a coarse grating, progressively finer stripes are presented. Acuity is taken as the finest stripe width to which the infant consistently responds according to the observer. Infants under 6 to 7 months of age show the same response pattern, even when visual stimulation is continued for 20 to 30 stimulus presentations. Infants older than 8 or 9 months of age need to be rewarded after each trial in order to keep their attention on the test situation. The test distance is 40cm for infants below 6 months of age, 57cm for infants between 6 and 12 months and 80cm for infants over 12 months.

In healthy term infants, grating acuity increases from 1 cycle per degree (c/deg) of visual angle at birth to 10c/deg at 52 weeks of age, with the greatest rate of development up to 5 months of age (Fig. 2.1). Grating acuity continues to improve throughout the first five years of life, with adult values being reached between 4 and 9 years (Teller *et al.* 1974, MacDonald *et al.* 1975, Atkinson *et al.* 1977, Dobson and Teller 1978, Gwiazda *et al.* 1980, Birch *et al.* 1983*a*, Lewis and Maurer 1986, Van Hof-van Duin and Mohn 1986*a*, Mohn *et al.* 1988, Heersema 1989). Acuity in low-risk preterm infants lags behind that of term infants up to the age of 6 to 8 months, and then reaches equal levels if age is calculated from birth. When age is corrected for preterm birth, acuities in the two groups are similar at all ages, but mean preterm acuity is consistently slightly higher than in the term infants (Van Hof-van Duin and Mohn 1986*a*).

Visual fields
Visual field size is assessed binocularly and monocularly using kinetic perimetry with an arc perimeter (Mohn and Van Hof-van Duin 1986). The apparatus consists of two 4cm wide black metal strips, mounted perpendicularly to each other and bent to form two arcs, each with a radius of 40cm. The perimeter is located in front of a black curtain concealing an observer who can watch the child's eye and head movements through a peephole.

The infant sits or is held in line with the centre of the arc perimeter. During fixation of a centrally positioned white ball, placed so as to subtend a visual angle of 6°, an identical target is slowly moved from the periphery towards the fixation point along one of the arcs of the perimeter. Eye and head movements toward the peripheral ball are used to estimate the border of the visual field. Orthogonal and oblique half-meridia are tested in a pseudo-random succession. The median of three measurements along each half-meridian is used as an estimate of the visual field size along that half-meridian.

The binocular visual field of the newborn extends to about 30° to either side along the horizontal meridian, while the vertical extent is only 15° above and 20° below the mid-point. The visual field shows little development between birth and 2 months of age, but expands rapidly until the age of 8 months, and more slowly until age 12 months (Fig. 2.2). By 12 months the upper visual field has reached the adult size, while the horizontal and lower fields reach adult values at around 15 months. The development of the monocular visual field in the temporal and vertical direction closely resembles that of the binocular field, but the nasal field is smaller than the temporal field at all ages and reaches adult values at 17 months (Heersema 1989, Heersema *et al.* 1989).

Optokinetic nystagmus (OKN)
OKN is the oculomotor response to the movement of a large patterned stimulus. The eye movements serve to stabilize the moving image of the world on the retina. Normally, OKN consists of slow eye movements in the direction of the stimulus movement, interrupted by fast saccadic movements in the opposite direction. OKN is tested by either recording or observing eye movements in response to the movement of a large field of randomly spaced 1cm dots to the right or to the left in

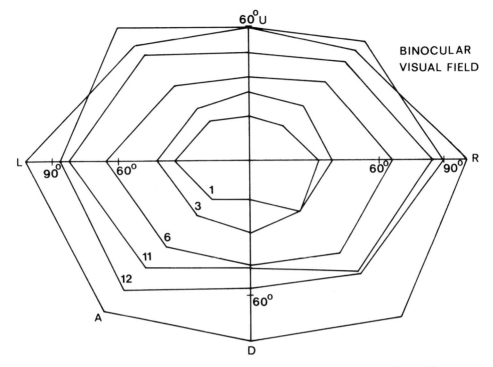

Fig. 2.2. Binocular visual field at age 1, 3, 6, 11 and 12 months. (L/R = left/right; U/D = up/down; A = adult field.)

front of the infant's head. For monocular testing, one eye is covered with an orthoptic eye-patch. Binocular OKN is normally directionally symmetrical from birth onwards, *i.e.* similar reactions are elicited by stimulation to the right and to the left. Visually impaired infants often show an asymmetrical binocular OKN, and usually asymmetries are related to the location of brain dysfunction as demonstrated with ultrasound or CT scans, with a poorer response to stimulation toward the damaged hemisphere (Van Hof-van Duin and Mohn 1983, 1986b, 1987; Groenendaal *et al.* 1989; Van Hof-van Duin *et al.* 1989). Monocular OKN (MOKN) is normally directionally asymmetrical from birth onwards, with a preference for temporal to nasal stimulation. MOKN is related to the development of binocular vision and becomes symmetrical by 4 months postnatally (Atkinson 1979, Van Hof-van Duin and Mohn 1984). In visually impaired and strabismic infants, the onset of symmetrical MOKN often is delayed or does not occur at all (Braddick and Atkinson 1983a; Van Hof-van Duin and Mohn 1986b, 1987; Van Hof-van Duin *et al.* 1987, 1989; Wattam-Bell *et al.* 1987; Groenendaal 1989).

Visual threat response
Defensive blinking, or the threat response (*i.e.* an eye blink in response to a rapidly

13

approaching object), consists of a tactile and a visual component. The tactile component is processed subcortically and is present in normal babies from birth onwards. The visual component is tested by holding a clear perspex sheet between the infant's eyes and the approaching object. Visual threat is processed cortically, and develops normally from 17 weeks after birth (Van Hof-van Duin and Mohn 1985, 1986*b*, 1987; Groenendaal *et al.* 1989; Van Hof-van Duin *et al.* 1989).

Age norms for grating acuity and visual field extension have been obtained in healthy term and preterm infants of 0 to 5 years of age (Van Hof-van Duin and Mohn 1984, 1985, 1986*a,b*; Mohn and Van Hof-van Duin 1986; Mohn *et al.* 1988; Heersema 1989; Heersema *et al.* 1989; Heersema and Van Hof-van Duin 1990; Van Hof-van Duin and Pott 1990). Development of grating acuity, visual fields, symmetrical monocular OKN and the visual component of the threat response of low risk preterm infants lies within the range of that of term infants of comparable conceptional rather than postnatal age. Little evidence of any beneficial effect of early extravisual experience has been found in low risk preterm infants (Kiff and Lepard 1966; Miranda 1970; Sokol and Joncs 1979; Dobson *et al.* 1980; Van Hof-van Duin *et al.* 1983; Van Hof-van Duin and Mohn 1984, 1985, 1987).

The various behavioural methods of assessing visual function have proved very useful for the assessment of visual development during the first years of life in infants at risk for neurological or developmental abnormalities and in visually impaired infants (Van Hof-van Duin and Mohn 1987).

Summary of findings in VLBW infants in Rotterdam study
Impaired visual development was demonstrated in 50 to 70 per cent of very low birthweight (VLBW, <1500g) infants during the first 12 months after expected term (Van Hof-van Duin *et al.* 1989). No single visual function appeared to be specifically susceptible to impairment. In fact, deficits were often apparent across a range of functions. Visual impairments could be assessed at 6 weeks corrected age, and the highest incidence of visual impairments was found at 6 months corrected age. Beyond 6 months fewer deficits were observed, which suggests that in many infants visual development is delayed rather than permanently impaired. In some infants, particularly in those with neurological impairments, visual deficits including strabismus become evident beyond 6 months of age, after an apparently normal initial development (Miranda 1970, Atkinson *et al.* 1977, Mohn and Van Hof-van Duin 1986). Longitudinal visual assessment of VLBW infants at 2½ and 5 years of age showed that visual impairments appeared to be rather constant, indicating that VLBW infants are indeed at risk for permanent visual impairments (Lewis and Maurer 1986, Heersema 1989).

Recently it has been demonstrated that perinatal hypoxia and preterm birth form a serious risk for abnormal visual development, with the highest incidence of visual impairments at 3 to 6 months of age (Groenendaal *et al.* 1989, Heersema 1989). Analysis of other perinatal risk factors is under study.

In terms of the four visual functions described above, it has become possible to

TABLE 2.1

Clinical assessment of vision

1. Discussion of child's medical/family history of visual problems

2. Observation of general visuomotor behaviour

3. Orthoptic tests

4. Acuity assessment:
   Forced-choice preferential looking (see text)
   STYCAR (Sheridan 1976)
   Sheridan–Gardiner (Sheridan 1970)
   Cambridge Crowding Cards (Atkinson *et al.* 1987*a*)

5. Photorefraction/videorefraction and retinoscopy

6. Binocular vision:
   Monocular optokinetic nystagmus
   Binocular visual evoked potential stereopsis, correlation

7. Discussion of results

detect visual impairments at early ages. Early detection of such impairments, followed by stimulation adapted to the specific deficit and the remaining visual capacity of the individual child, may well be valuable and helpful in preventing disturbances in further visuomotor and cognitive development. Considering the developmental course of visual functions in children at risk for visual impairment, the age recommended for visual assessment is around 6 to 7 months. Re-examination at later ages is needed to substantiate the diagnosis of a visual defect and/or to determine whether visual development is progressing.

Visual assessment in Cambridge, UK

Over the past 15 years the Visual Development Unit, University of Cambridge, has built up a repertoire of assessment methods in research and has adapted them for vision assessment in clinical paediatric patients and in groups where there is a high risk of visual defect.

Children assessed in the Unit vary a great deal along both dichotomies outlined above (mild/severe disability and visual only/MHVI). This means that the tests have to be adaptable for a range of development from the normal to the severely neurologically impaired and for children with and without accompanying behavioural, motor, cognitive and emotional problems.

Several years ago a battery of tests (Table 2.1) was devised in Cambridge to assess acuity, binocularity, refraction, focusing ability and attention. Several other tests were included for assessment of specific subgroups (*e.g.* field testing in children with hemiplegia). The varied population of referrals was classified by age and diagnosis (Table 2.2). Over three quarters of this cohort had at least one visual defect (Table 2.3). A general description of the tests used has already been published (Atkinson 1985, 1986, 1989*a*) and so will not be described in detail here.

15

TABLE 2.2

Clinical referrals* for visual assessment to Visual Development Unit, Cambridge, Jan. 1983–Dec. 1984 (N = 108): age groups and diagnoses

Age group		
4 months–4 years	100	(developmental age generally under 2 years)
5–12 years	8	

Paediatric diagnosis	
Global developmental delay	33
Cerebral palsy	32
Down syndrome	6
Respiratory distress syndrome at preterm birth	6
Infantile convulsions	6
Language/speech/reading delay	5
Post-traumatic episode	4
Microcephaly	2
Dysmorphic syndrome	2
Others†	12

*30% of referrals were because of a known or strongly suspected visual disorder; 70% were for general visual assessment without any prior diagnosis of any visual problem.

†Other diagnoses included one each of: prenatal muscular atrophy; spina bifida; microphthalmia; hydrocephaly; hypothyroid function; macrocephaly; Prader–Willi syndrome; Rubenstein–Taybi syndrome; Sturge–Weber syndrome; chromosome abnormality (not Down syndrome); retinopathy of prematurity; extensive intracranial haemorrhage.

TABLE 2.3

Outcome of visual assessments (N = 108)

Abnormality	N	%
Visual acuity/amblyopia	49	45
Strabismus/abnormal eye movements	50	46
Poor visual attention/perceptual deficit	51	47
Abnormal refraction under cycloplegia	48	44
'Cortical blindness'—no confirmed ocular pathology	12	11
Confirmed ocular pathology	4	4
(Visual field deficit	9/12)	
Total with one or more visual defects	87	81

Assessment of acuity

In general the forced choice preferential looking (FPL) method used in Cambridge is very similar to that used in the Rotterdam study (see above). The main difference is that the Cambridge FPL acuity set-up is automated and fixed in position with the stripe patterns electronically displayed (Atkinson *et al.* 1977, 1982, 1986; Atkinson and Braddick 1982a). The observer is 'forced' to choose at the end of each presentation the side the child 'preferred' and to make his or her choice 'blind' (a microcomputer generates a random sequence of pattern presentation on the left or right monitor for each trial). The advantages of this automated version are speed of testing and elimination of possible observer bias. The disadvantage in comparison with the manual card system are its fixed position, making it suitable only for a clinical unit, and its relative cost.

Isotropic photorefraction and videorefraction

Photorefraction and videorefraction have been used extensively, both with and without cycloplegia, to measure focusing ability (which can also be used as an indicator of changes in visual attention) and refractive errors. Details of the isotropic technique and the results of its use in screening are described elsewhere (Atkinson and Braddick 1982*b*; Howland *et al.* 1983; Atkinson *et al.* 1984, 1987*b*; Braddick and Atkinson 1984; Braddick *et al.* 1988). The screening studies have allowed the course of emmetropization to be studied in children from birth to 5 years. In general, in terms of non-cycloplegic focus (*i.e.* free accommodation) newborns demonstrate a wide range of focus with the mean tending to be a small degree of myopia. Infants over 6 months improve their ability to change focus and to accommodate accurately to targets at different distances (Braddick *et al.* 1979), although over 50 per cent of normal infants show some astigmatism (Howland *et al.* 1978, Atkinson *et al.* 1987*b*). The incidence of astigmatism falls to adult levels by 2 years of age (Atkinson *et al.* 1980). By 6 to 9 months, accommodation is reasonably accurate although focusing tends on average to be slightly myopic in dim illumination (dark focus). The mean cycloplegic refraction is hyperopic at birth. The mean cycloplegic refraction (of the lower hypermetropic meridian) is around 1D hypermetropic in the majority of children at 9 months of age. Hypermetropia under cycloplegia of over 2D, beyond 1 year of age, places the child at risk for strabismus and amblyopia (Ingram *et al.* 1979, Braddick *et al.* 1988, Atkinson 1993). In general, emmetropization is rapid over the first two years of life, with many children reaching adult cycloplegic refractions (having lost their initial astigmatism) by 2 years of age.

Isotropic photorefraction has been used in the Cambridge Infant Screening Programme (Atkinson *et al.* 1987*b*, Atkinson 1993) to identify infants at risk for strabismus and amblyopia. In this programme a randomized control trial was conducted in which spectacles were worn in infancy to correct excessive degrees of hypermetropia (long-sightedness) and anisometropia (over 1D difference of refraction between the eyes). Subjects were identified at 6 to 9 months of age, and were followed up at four-month intervals to 4½ years. Without correction, 70 per cent of the 4-year-olds who had severe hypermetropia in infancy showed visual deficits (strabismus and/or amblyopia) compared to 25 per cent of the children with similar degrees of hypermetropia in infancy who had worn spectacles to partially correct their refractive errors in infancy. The mechanisms underlying this potentially valuable intervention are not clearly understood: neither conventional models of accommodative strabismus nor uniocular amblyopia fit the data well. We hypothesize that infant vision screening may identify not only children with refractive errors, who are at risk for strabismus and amblyopia, but also a subset of children with mild global developmental delay. If this is the case, it may have implications for understanding the precursors of certain learning disabilities such as dyslexia.

Cycloplegic videorefraction used in clinical assessment enables the tester to gauge whether the refraction of a clinical patient is in line with that of a normal child of the same age. Amblyopia can also be measured in isolation from refractive defocus by measuring acuity with and without spectacles (to correct any refractive errors). If acuity is in the normal range when correcting spectacles are worn then the child can be said to be non-amblyopic. However, estimates of amblyopia from FPL tests should be viewed with caution, as they often underestimate amblyopia compared to measures of recognition acuity.

Videorefraction can also be used without cycloplegia to monitor switches of visual attention between objects at different distances. Normal newborn infants tend to attend visually (and to focus) in relatively nearby space, and do not relax their accommodation sufficiently for targets beyond 1m distance. Infants over 6 months can extend their focus to at least 1.5m when attending to objects of interest. Many neurological paediatric patients show abnormal patterns of change of visual attention measured in this way (Atkinson 1989a). For example, many children with cerebral palsy show fixed focus either at near distances (similar to newborns) or at a similar position to their cycloplegic refraction. Some Down syndrome children focus in nearby space in a similar way to normal young infants (although their cycloplegic refraction may be in the normal hypermetropic range).

Clinically speaking, videorefraction is a very useful technique in that it is easy to learn and to carry out, it compares well with retinoscopy, and it is fast, reliable, safe and transportable. There is a family of theoretically related photorefractive techniques (Braddick and Atkinson 1984, Howland 1991) each of which has certain advantages and disadvantages. Use of a combination of these methods will probably turn out to be an optimal strategy for clinical assessment.

Indicators of cortical vision
Current models of human visual development (Atkinson 1984, 1989b, 1992; Atkinson and Braddick 1990) propose different postnatal time scales for functioning of specific cortical pathways. Each cortical stream processes information for different visual attributes or combinations of attributes. Onset of channels responsible for carrying information on binocularity, orientation discrimination, and mechanisms controlling visual selective attention are all thought to necessitate cortical functioning. Using these concepts, a number of 'designer' stimuli have been developed in the Visual Development Unit to dissociate subcortical from cortical visual systems. To illustrate how these tests can be used to demonstrate cortical function and developmental plasticity, studies on four paediatric subgroups are

briefly described below. The four groups are:

A—infants with a first degree relative with strabismus and/or amblyopia (Wattam-Bell *et al.* 1987);

B—infants with early onset strabismus (Smith *et al.* 1989, Atkinson *et al.* 1991*b*);

C—children with multiple disabilities including possible attentional losses (Hood and Atkinson 1990);

D—a subset of preterm VLBW infants with or without intraventricular haemorrhages (Atkinson *et al.* 1991*a*).

As details of the tests have been published elsewhere they will only be outlined here.

GROUP A: INFANTS WITH A FIRST DEGREE RELATIVE WITH STRABISMUS AND/OR AMBLYOPIA

The interaction of inputs from the two eyes is a property of the majority of striate cortical cells but is not found in earlier (subcortical) stages of visual processing. This interaction registers any disparities between the two images. Stereoscopic vision is absent or poor in strabismic individuals, cortical cells becoming dominated during development by inputs from the non-strabismic eye.

Two techniques (VEP recordings to random dot correlograms and stereograms, and FPL procedures to the same patterns) have been used to assess the development of binocular vision in normal infants (*e.g.* Braddick *et al.* 1979, 1983; Fox 1981; Birch *et al.* 1983*b*, 1985; Braddick and Atkinson 1983*b*). An alternative measure of binocularity is that of the symmetry of monocular OKN, described above. In general, the age at onset of binocular VEP and that of symmetrical OKN are similar (Braddick and Atkinson 1983*a*).

In the Cambridge study (Wattam-Bell *et al.* 1987), a group of infants at risk for strabismus because of their family history (*i.e.* infants with at least one first degree relative who had been strabismic and/or amblyopic in childhood) were tested longitudinally to discern the onset of binocularity, as demonstrated by a significant VEP to a correlogram and symmetrical OKN responses. Most normal children develop disparity detection by the age of 4 months. This was also found to hold true for most of the study group. The correlation between the age at onset of the correlogram VEP and OKN symmetry was significant but weak, and some infants showed early OKN symmetry but no binocular VEP. The results suggest that OKN does not depend on exactly the same neural substrate as the VEP response.

In total, 9.5 per cent of the 105 at-risk children became strabismic. One or two infants became strabismic before 4 months and so did not show the binocular VEP response (although this could have been due to eye misalignment at the time of testing). In several children normal binocularity developed initially but became disrupted by later onset strabismus. The results indicate that these strabismic children did not lack the necessary prerequisites for developing this aspect of cortical function early in life, but that some other factor precipitating the strabismus had interfered with the normal course of development. There was a significant increase in ammetropia in the cycloplegic refractions of the strabismus history group at 9 months of age compared to the normal population (Anker *et al.* 1991).

GROUP B: INFANTS WITH EARLY ONSET STRABISMUS

Similar tests to those described above have been used to measure binocularity in infants who became strabismic before the age of 6 months (Smith *et al.* 1989, Atkinson *et al.* 1991*b*), together with longitudinal monocular acuity testing using FPL, refractive measures using videorefraction, retinoscopy and standard tests of stereopsis at 4 years of age (Frisby *et al.* 1975, Saye and Frisby 1975, Walraven 1975, Okuda *et al.* 1977, Lang 1983). These children were tested before and after surgery to realign the eyes (surgery taking place before 2 years of age).

Some children demonstrated stereoscopic vision by detecting a relatively large disparity (40′) when tested with FPL stereograms in the months just before and immediately after surgery. There was some overall improvement in binocular status for the entire group after surgery. This result suggests an extraordinary range of cortical plasticity in the first two years of life both for developing disparity detectors initially (to accommodate large angles of anomalous correspondence) and for retuning these mechanisms after surgery, when the eyes have been aligned. However, on testing at 4 years of age (two years after surgery), very few of these same children had any stereoscopic vision, and those who did responded only to relatively coarse disparities on the standard clinical stereo tests. It appears as if their original tenuous stereopsis had been lost (although the surgical realignment was good, being within 10 prism diopters). It is possible that better final binocularity would have been obtained if the surgical realignment had been done even earlier, but until control studies are carried out comparing late and early surgery this must remain hypothetical.

In spite of relatively early surgery, refractive correction, and occlusion therapy prescribed before surgery (and in some cases also after surgery), many of these children showed small degrees of amblyopia when tested at 4 years (acuity being measured with the Cambridge Crowding Cards—Atkinson *et al.* 1987*a*). On monocular FPL immediately before and after surgery there was on average an improvement in acuity, with reduced interocular differences postoperatively. However, many of the infants showed only relatively small or no interocular differences, even before surgery. It was also noted that many of these children had abnormal refractions on retinoscopy (moderate to high levels of hypermetropia and anisometropia under cycloplegia) through the first two years of life.

The results of this study suggest high degrees of plasticity in development of binocular systems to allow development of disparity detectors even though the eyes are not well aligned. They also cast doubt on the belief that good binocularity (normal levels of stereo acuity) can be developed in children with early onset strabismus following surgery in the first two years of life; any early binocularity seems to be reduced or lost by 4 years. In addition, although dense amblyopia is relatively rare in this group with early intervention, and for the group as a whole

TABLE 2.4

Numbers of children completing behavioural and electrophysiological tasks (clinical group vs. comparison 1- and 3-month-olds)*

Group	+FS/+VEP	+FS/−VEP	−FS/+VEP	−FS/−VEP
Normal 1-month-olds (N = 18)	4	14	0	0
Normal 3-month-olds (N = 14)	12	2	0	0
Clinical group (see text) (N = 15)	2	5	3	5

*Adapted by permission from Hood and Atkinson (1990).
Behavioural testing involved observing fixation shift (FS) response in non-competition and competition conditions. In non-competition (NC), only one target for fixation is visible at any one time: when the central target is switched off, the laterally peripheral target is switched on. In competition (C), both targets are visible simultaneously and compete for the child's attention.
+FS/−FS: ⩾8/<8 out of 10 correct refixations in NC and C conditions.
+VEP/−VEP: positive/negative visual evoked potential at 1st, 2nd and 4th harmonics.

interocular differences were smaller after surgery than before, this study does not indicate whether this would also have been the case with much later surgery. Further studies with both early and late surgery, and detailed measures of occlusion compliance, are needed before these questions can be answered.

GROUP C: CHILDREN WITH MULTIPLE DISABILITIES INCLUDING POSSIBLE ATTENTIONAL LOSSES: DISSOCIATION OF SENSORY VISUAL LOSS FROM ATTENTIONAL LOSS
The ability to make rapid saccades to position a laterally peripheral target on the fovea underlies perimetry and field testing discussed in the Rotterdam studies. Newborn infants are found to have an additional problem, indicated by a reduction in field size, if a central target remains visible when the peripheral target appears (Harris and MacFarlane 1974; MacFarlane et al. 1976; Atkinson and Braddick 1985; Atkinson et al. 1988a, 1990; Braddick and Atkinson 1988). Even when the targets are matched across 1- and 3-month-olds for contrast sensitivity (just above contrast threshold), the younger infants show longer latencies to refixate when there is competition between a central and a peripheral target.

Mechanisms for shifting visual attention are thought to involve both subcortical (superior colliculus) and cortical (parietal lobes, frontal eye fields) circuitry (Mountcastle 1978, Hyvarinen 1982, Schiller 1985, Andersen 1988, Posner and Rothbart 1990). Deficits in selective attention have been found in patients with parietal lobe damage and in primates with damage to the frontal eye fields. For example, patients with Balint syndrome, involving bilateral parietal damage, have great difficulty in disengaging attention from one object of interest to attend to another (De Renzi 1982). This deficit is similar to the behaviour in 1-month-olds when viortical (superg stimuli.

In this study a subgroup of children referred to the Visual Development Unit were tested for ability to fixate a target under conditions of competition and non-competition (Table 2.4). The criterion for inclusion was that the child had previously shown significant VEPs to either a pattern reversal or a pattern onset stimulus in central vision, yet on informal testing did not appear to have spontaneous visual searching. In order to exclude those with severe motor apraxia, only children who were capable of consistently fixing and tracking a large coloured toy or pen-light moved slowly from the midline to the periphery were included. These children were compared on a fixation shift task with groups of normal 1- and 3-month-olds. A phase reversing grating pattern of high contrast black and white bars was used as the stimulus. The black and white bars alternate over time at a given repetition rate. Peripheral VEPs were recorded in the same eccentricity and with the same stimuli as used in the fixation shift task (phase reversing at 6 repetitons per second (rps), low spatial frequency vertical bar pattern, 50 per cent contrast). Table 2.4 shows the number of children in each group who showed a significant peripheral VEP and refixated the peripheral target correctly. Nearly all of the 3-month-olds showed a significant VEP to this pattern in the periphery and consistently refixated the peripheral target in both the competition and non-competition conditions. Most 1-month-olds showed accurate refixations but did not produce a significant peripheral VEP. Some of the clinical group behaved like the 1-month-olds and others like the 3-month-olds. However, three of the clinical group children showed a significant peripheral VEP, indicating that the incoming sensory pathways were intact, but did not actively refixate the target in either the non-competition or competition conditions. This would indicate a possible dissociation in these children between sensory and attentional mechanisms. Further research using modifications of this type of paradigm may enable us to categorize attentional deficits more finely. However, care will need to be taken regarding spatiotemporal tuning to enable the optimum stimuli to be used.

GROUP D: PRETERM VLBW INFANTS

The cortex possesses channels specifically tuned to different orientations (Hubel and Wiesel 1977). This sensitivity is not found in subcortical systems. A paradigm used to test for the presence of orientation-selective channels has been designed. This consists of analysing a VEP to a sinusoidal grating pattern, which alternates between two oblique orientations separated by 90° (Braddick *et al.* 1986; Atkinson *et al.* 1987c, 1988b; Braddick and Atkinson 1988). This paradigm has been used to monitor the development of orientation sensitivity with age. For relatively slow alternation rates (3rps) the orientation response is found shortly after birth, while for more rapid alternation the response emerges around 6 weeks of age. The response is both temporally and spatially tuned (Atkinson *et al.* 1989a).

As cortical visual function may be a good indicator of the general state of neurological development, this orientation measure has been used to investigate development in a high risk group: a volunteer cohort of preterm VLBW infants (Atkinson *et al.* 1991a). This group was matched for gestational age with a group of control infants, and five different tests were compared across the two groups: (1) orientation reversal VEP at 5 and 13 weeks of age; (2) phase reversal VEP at 5 and

TABLE 2.5

**Clinical referrals to Visual Development Unit, Cambridge,
Jan. 1990–Dec. 1991 (N = 110; ages mainly 0–5 years)**

	%
Paediatric diagnosis	
Ophthalmological problem only	11
Cerebral palsy	31
Other neurological disabilities	58
(focal lesions	5)
Outcome of visual assessment	
Abnormal eye movements—strabismus/nystagmus	77
Reduced acuity	74
Abnormal cycloplegic refraction	69
Poor accommodative control on videorefraction	61
Absence of fine visuomotor coordination	46

13 weeks; (3) fixation shift test at 4 to 5 weeks, as described above; (4) FPL acuity at 12 to 13 weeks and at 28 weeks; (5) cyclopegic videorefraction at 6 to 8 months.

In summary, no difference was found between the groups on FPL acuity estimates or on accommodative ability measured using videorefraction, nor on any of the VEP measures. However, the VLBW group showed shorter latencies than the controls for refixating saccadically a peripheral target. This suggests that the development of control mechanisms for visuomotor tasks of this kind may well be sensitive to the extent of visual experience. Current models of selective attention would suggest that collicular–parietal processing is involved in these responses, whereas acuity and orientation specificity may reflect the maturation of the geniculostriate pathway. These data may be used to investigate differential critical periods related to different processing streams in human visual development, and to assess neurological delays in at-risk infants.

In comparison with the Rotterdam studies on preterm infants it should be noted that the small group studied in Cambridge comprised babies volunteered by their parents and who were therefore likely to be in a generally healthier state than many of their contemporaries within the special care baby nursery. It is also worth noting that one recent study has estimated that only 15 per cent of VLBW infants will develop severe neurological problems (SPORU 1991), and that the Cambridge VLBW group constituted approximately only one third of all VLBW infants born in the Cambridge area within the recruiting period for this study.

General clinical assessments

A summary of Cambridge assessments over the past two years is given in Table 2.5. The main point to note is that, in the main, only the severely neurologically impaired group within the total paediatric clinical population is referred for visual assessments. Many of these children have common visual problems (strabismus,

23

TABLE 2.6

Atkinson Battery of Child Development for Examining Functional Vision (ABCDEFV): tests for infants up to 6 months

Tests performed at community clinic	Tests performed at assessment unit
Newborn (0–1 month)	
1. Pupil response 2. Diffuse light reaction 3. Intermittent tracking 4. Videorefraction	1. OKN 2. VEP (PA and PR)* 3. FLP 4. Videorefraction
1–3 months	
1. Onset of smiling to face 2. Improved tracking (3/5 successful trials) 3. Convergence to approach 4. Peripheral refixation in blank field 5. Videorefraction	1. OKN 2. VEP (PA and PR)* 3. Orientation reversal VEP 4. FPL 5. Fixation shifts (attention) 6. Videorefraction
4–6 months	
1. Good saccadic tracking 2. Batting (waving arm at target), followed by reach 3. Follows retreat to 3m 4. Tracking behind barrier 5. Defensive blink reliable 6. Regards hands, then feet 7. Responds to visual 'peekaboo' 8. Peripheral refixation to face 9. No squint 10. Watches object fall in visual field 11. Retrieves partially covered object 12. Videorefraction	1. FPL acuity 3c/deg or better 2. Orientation reversal VEP 3. Videorefraction—focus changes 4. Stereo VEP and FPL 5. OKN symmetry 6. Fixation shifts and competition

*PA—pattern appearance/disappearance; PR—phase reversal of pattern stimulus.

poor acuity, refractive errors) and many show poor control of accommodation and fixation shifts, indicating abnormal attentional mechanisms in addition to deficits of sensory and perceptual vision.

The need for tests of functional vision

From the results of the above assessments, details can be given of the visual orthoptic and ophthalmological status of the child. However, one of the major problems with multiply impaired children is understanding their visual defects in terms of implied 'disability' and understanding the interactive effects of visual defects with other paediatric problems. What is needed is a functional test of vision which will provide information on which particular everyday tasks will be impeded by the visual defects assessed. At present very few paediatric studies have been published which address these problems. In addition, most of the tests described are only concerned with brain mechanisms involved with the initial analysis of

TABLE 2.7

Examination of visual tracking in newborn infants

Test conditions
- Five trials, on separate occasions, within 30 minutes of waking
- Target: 5cm, high contrast object (*e.g.* Christmas bauble)—10° at 30cm viewing distance
- Velocity: 5°/s, 10°/s (2.5cm/s, 5cm/s)
- Movement from midline, local movement allowed
- Body support (head/neck) in semi-supine position

Expected result
- 1/5 or 2/5 successes with saccadic tracking 15–20° from midline
- Occasional head movements following eye movements
- Long latency for both eye and head movements (several seconds)

visual stimuli into component parts. Perceptual analysis must be used to put these attributes together to recognize objects, to separate them from their background, to categorize them and to initiate appropriate actions. This means that tests of perceptuocognitive and perceptuomotor vision must be included in visual assessments.

As a preliminary attempt to address some of these problems, the Visual Development Unit has drawn up a list of tests with appropriate protocols for different age groups, combining ideas from the present assessments in vision, established paediatric tests (*e.g.* Sheridan–Gardiner—Sheridan 1970), and ideas from developmental psychology (Piagetian object permanence tasks, spatial representation and construction tasks). The battery is called the Atkinson Battery of Child Development for Examining Functional Vision (ABCDEFV) (Atkinson *et al.* 1989*b*). An outline of part of it is shown in Table 2.6. Each test willl have a defined protocol so that the procedures are standardized across testers (an example relating to tracking in newborn infants is shown in Table 2.7). This is to avoid the obvious problems of misunderstanding based on clinical procedures such as 'fixes and follows', where there is a general notion as to what this phrase means clinically but no easily defined 'pass' or 'failure' criterion by which to judge an individual child's visual behaviour against normal behaviour.

The battery is divided into two sections. The first contains tests which are portable, relate to everyday living, and can be carried out in the home, the community clinic or the clinician's private office. The other comprises tasks which require specialist equipment (mainly non-portable) and, in many cases, specialist skills: these should be conducted in a specialized unit or hospital clinic. At present the battery is being normalized for each age group. It is inevitable that in this process some tests will need to be modified if they are going to prove reliable and informative, and some may eventually be eliminated.

There are still many other aspects of funtional vision for which assessment methods have yet to be designed. In developing the ABCDEFV it is hoped eventually to define the limitations of blind and partially sighted children of different ages and to devise more effective treatment, rehabilitation and educational methods, especially for the multiply impaired. Assessment of infant vision has advanced considerably over the past 15 years, but much research remains to be done before we can answer fully all the questions that have been posed.

ACKNOWLEDGMENTS

These studies were supported by the Medical Research Council of Great Britain, the Wellcome Trust and the East Anglia Regional Health Authority (Cambridge) and by the Praeventiefonds, 's-Gravenhage, the Netherlands (Rotterdam).

REFERENCES

Anker, S., Atkinson, J., Bobier, W., Tricklebank, J., Wattam-Bell, J. (1991) 'Infant vision screening programme: can early detection of refractive errors in infants with a family history of strabismus predict later visual problems?' *Proceedings of the 7th International Orthoptic Congress, Nuremberg. (Abstract 154.)*

Andersen, R.A. (1988) 'The neurological basis of spatial cognition: role of the parietal lobe.' *In:* Stiles-Davis, J., Kritchevsky, M., Bellugi, U. (Eds) *Spatial Cognition: Brain Bases and Development.* Hillsdale, NJ: Laurence Erlbaum, pp. 57–80.

Atkinson, J. (1979) 'Development of optokinetic nystagmus in the human infant and infant monkey: an analogue to development in kittens.' *In:* Freeman, R.D. (Ed.) *Developmental Neurobiology of Vision.* New York: Plenum, pp. 277–287.

—— (1984) 'Human visual development over the first six months of life. A review and a hypothesis.' *Human Neurobiology,* **3,** 61–74.

—— (1985) 'Assessment of vision in infants and young children.' *In:* Harel, S, Anastasiow, N.J. (Eds) *The At-Risk Infant: Psycho/Socio/Medical Aspects.* Baltimore: Paul H. Brookes, pp. 341–352.

—— (1986) 'Methods of objective assessment of visual functions in subjects with limited communication skills.' *In:* Ellis, D. (Ed.) *Sensory Impairment in Mentally Handicapped People.* Beckenham, Kent: Croom Holm, pp. 201–217.

—— (1989a) 'New tests of vision screening and assessment in infants and young children.' *In:* French, J.H., Harel, S., Casaer, P. (Eds) *Child Neurology and Developmental Disabilities.* Baltimore: Paul H. Brookes, pp. 219–227.

—— (1989b) 'Subcortical or cortical control of newborn vision? A revised model.' *Ophthalmic and Physiological Optics,* **9,** 469. *(Abstract.)*

—— (1992) 'Early visual development: differential functioning of parvocellular and magnocellular pathways.' *Eye,* **6,** 129–135.

—— (1993) 'Infant vision screening: prediction and prevention of strabismus and amblyopia from refractive screening in the Cambridge photorefraction programme.' *In:* Simons, K. (Ed.) *Early Visual Development: Normal and Abnormal.* New York: Oxford University Press. *(In press.)*

—— Braddick, O.J. (1982a) 'Assessment of visual acuity in infancy and early childhood.' *Acta Ophthalmologica,* **157** (Suppl.), 18–26.

—— —— (1982b) 'The use of isotropic photorefraction for vision screening in infants.' *Acta Ophthalmologica,* **157** (Suppl.), 36–45.

—— —— (1985) 'Early development of the control of visual attention.' *Perception,* **14,** A25. *(Abstract.)*

—— —— (1990) 'The developmental course of cortical processing streams in the human infant.' *In:* Blakemore, C. (Ed.) *Vision: Coding and Efficiency.* Cambridge: Cambridge University Press, 247–253.

—— —— Moar, K. (1977) 'Development of contrast sensitivity over the first three months of life in the human infant.' *Vision Research,* **17,** 1037—1044.

—— —— French, J. (1980) 'Infant astigmatism: its disappearance with age.' *Vision Research,* **20,** 891–893.

—— —— Pimm-Smith, E. (1982) 'Preferential looking for monocular and binocular acuity testing of infants.' *British Journal of Ophthalmology*, **66**, 264–268.

—— —— Durden, K., Watson, P.G., Atkinson, S. (1984) 'Screening for refractive errors in 6–9 months old infants by photorefraction.' *British Journal of Ophthalmology*, **68**, 105–112.

—— Wattam-Bell, J., Pimm-Smith, E., Evans, C., Braddick, O.J. (1986) 'Comparison of rapid procedures in forced choice preferential looking for estimating acuity in infants and young children.' *Documenta Ophthalmologica Proceedings Series*, **45**, 192–200.

—— Anker, S., Evans, C., McIntyre, A. (1987a) 'The Cambridge Crowding Cards for preschool visual acuity testing.' *In: Transactions of the 6th International Orthoptic Congress, Harrogate, England.*

—— Braddick, O.J., Wattam-Bell, J., Durden, K., Bobier, W., Pointer, J., Atkinson, S. (1987b) 'Photorefractive screening of infants and effects of refractive correction.' *Investigative Ophthalmology and Visual Science*, **28** (Suppl.), 399. *(Abstract.)*

—— Hood, B., Wattam-Bell, J. (1987c), 'Discrimination by infants of orientation in dynamic patterns.' *Perception*, **16**, 232. *(Abstract.)*

—— —— Braddick, O.J., Wattam-Bell, J. (1988a) 'Infants' control of fixation shifts with single and competing targets: mechanisms of shifting attention.' *Perception*, **17**, 367–368.

—— —— Wattam-Bell, J., Anker, S., Tricklebank, J. (1988b) 'Development of orientation discrimination in infancy.' *Perception*, **17**, 587–595.

—— Braddick, O.J., Wattam-Bell, J., Hood, B., Weeks, F (1989a) 'Temporal frequency and orientation selectivity of young infants' orientation-specific responses.' *Ophthalmic and Physiological Optics*, **9**, 468. *(Abstract.)*

—— Gardner, N., Tricklebank, J., Anker, S. (1989b) 'Atkinson Battery of Child Development for Examining Functional Vision (ABCDEFV).' *Ophthalmic and Physiological Optics*, **9**, 470. *(Abstract.)*

—— Braddick, O.J., Weeks, F., Hood, B. (1990) 'Spatial and temporal tuning of infants' orientation-specific responses.' *Perception*, **19**, 371. *(Abstract.)*

—— —— Anker, S., Hood, B., Wattam-Bell, J., Weeks, F., Rennie, J., Coughtrey, H. (1991a) 'Visual development in the VLBW infant.' *Transactions of the 3rd Meeting of the Child Vision Research Society, Rotterdam.*

—— Smith, J., Anker, S., Wattam-Bell, J., Braddick, O.J., Moore, A.T. (1991b) 'Binocularity and amblyopia before and after early strabismus surgery.' *Investigative Ophthalmological and Visual Science*, **32**, 820. *(Abstract.)*

Birch, E.E., Gwiazda, J., Bauer, J.A., Nagele, J., Held, R. (1983a) 'Visual acuity and its meridional variations in children aged 7–60 months.' *Vision Research*, **23**, 1019–1024.

—— —— Held, R. (1983b) 'The development of vergence does not account for the development of stereopsis.' *Perception*, **12**, 331–336.

—— Shimojo, S., Held, R. (1985) 'Preferential-looking assessment of fusion and stereopsis in infants aged 1–6 months.' *Investigative Ophthalmology and Visual Science*, **26**, 366–370.

Braddick, O.J., Atkinson, J. (1983a) 'Some recent findings on the development of human binocularity: a review.' *Behavioural Brain Research*, **10**, 141–150.

—— —— (1983b) 'Stimulus control in VEP and behavioural assessment of infant vision.' *Annals of the New York Academy of Sciences*, **388**, 642–644.

—— —— (1984) 'Photorefractive techniques: applications in testing infants and young children.' *In: Transactions of the 1st International Congress of the British College of Ophthalmic Opticians (Optometrists), Vol. 2*, pp. 26–34.

—— —— (1988) 'Sensory selectivity attentional control, and cross-channel integration in early visual development.' *In: Yonas, A. (Ed.) 20th Minnesota Symposium on Child Psychology.* Hillsdale, NJ: Lawrence Erlbaum, pp. 105–143.

—— —— French, J., Howland, H.C. (1979) 'A photo-refractive study of infant accommodation.' *Vision Research*, **19**, 319–330.

—— Wattam-Bell, J., Day, J., Atkinson, J. (1983) 'The onset of binocular function in human infants.' *Human Neurobiology*, **2**, 65–69.

—— —— —— (1986) 'Orientation-specific cortical responses develop in early infancy.' *Nature*, **320**, 617–619.

—— Atkinson, J., Wattam-Bell, J., Anker, S., Norris, V. (1988) 'Videorefractive screening of accommodative performance in infants.' *Investigative Ophthalmology and Visual Science*, **29** (Suppl.), 60. *(Abstract.)*

De Renzi, E. (1982) 'Oculomotor disturbances in hemispheric disease.' *In:* Johnston, C.W., Pirozzolo, F.J. (Eds.) *Neuropsychology of Eye Movements.* Hillsdale, NJ: Lawrence Erlbaum, pp. 177–200.

Dobson, V., Teller, D.Y. (1978) 'Visual acuity in human infants: a review and comparison of behavioural and electrophysiological studies.' *Vision Research*, **18**, 1469–1483.

—— Mayer, D.L., Lee, C.P. (1980) 'Visual acuity screening of preterm infants.' *Investigative Ophthalmology and Visual Science*, **19**, 1498–1505.

Fox, R. (1981) 'Stereopsis in animals and human infants.' *In:* Aslin, R.N., Alberts, J.R., Petersen, M.R. (Eds) *The Development of Perception: Psychobiological Perspectives. Vol. 2: The Visual System.* New York: Academic Press, pp. 335–381.

Frisby, J.P., Mein, J., Saye, A., Stanworth, A. (1975) 'Use of random dot stereograms in the clinical assessment of strabismic patients.' *British Journal of Ophthalmology*, **59**, 545–552.

Groenendaal, F., Van Hof-van Duin, J., Baerts, W., Fetter, W.P.F. (1989) 'Effects of perinatal hypoxia on visual development during the first year of (corrected) age.' *Early Human Development*, **20**, 267–279.

Gwiazda, J., Brill, S., Mohindra, L., Held, R. (1980) 'Preferential looking acuity in infants from two to fifty-eight weeks of age.' *American Journal of Optometry and Physiological Optics*, **57**, 428–432.

Harris, P.L., MacFarlane, A. (1974) 'The growth of the effective visual field from birth to seven weeks.' *Journal of Experimental Psychology*, **18**, 340–384.

Heersema, D.J. (1989) *Perinatale Risicofactoren en Viseuele Ontwikkeling bij Jonge Kinderen.* Rotterdam: Erasmus Universiteits Drukkerij. (PhD thesis.)

—— Van Hof-van Duin, J. (1990) 'Age norms for visual acuity in toddlers using the acuity card procedure.' *Clinical Vision Sciences*, **5**, 167–174.

—— —— Hop, W.C.J. (1989) 'Age norms for visual field development in children aged 0 to 4 years using arc perimetry.' *Investigative Ophthalmology and Visual Science*, **30** (Suppl.), 242. *(Abstract.)*

Hood, B., Atkinson, J. (1990) 'Sensory visual loss and cognitive deficits in the selective attentional system of normal infants and neurologically impaired children.' *Developmental Medicine and Child Neurology*, **32**, 1067–1077.

Howland, H.C. (1991) 'Advances in instrumentation for biometry of infant refractive error.' *Investigative Ophthalmology and Visual Science*, **32** (Suppl.), xii. *(Abstract.)*

—— Atkinson, J., Braddick, O.J., French, J. (1978) 'Infant astigmatism measured by photorefraction.' *Science*, **202**, 331–333.

—— Braddick, O.J., Atkinson, J., Howland, B. (1983) 'Optics of photorefraction: orthogonal and isotropic methods.' *Journal of the Optical Society of America*, **73**, 1701–1708.

Hubel, D.R., Wiesel, T.N. (1977) 'Functional architecture of macaque monkey visual cortex.' *Proceedings of the Royal Society of London, Series B: Biological Sciences*, **198**, 1–59.

Hyvarinen, L. (1982) *The Parietal Cortex of Monkey and Man.* Berlin: Springer-Verlag.

Ingram, R.M. Traynar, M.J., Walker, C., Wilson, J.M. (1979) 'Screening for refractive errors at age 1 year: a pilot study.' *British Journal of Ophthalmology*, **63**, 243–250.

Kiff, R.D., Lepard, C. (1966) 'Visual response of premature infants.' *Archives of Ophthalmology*, **75**, 631–633.

Lang, J. (1983) 'A new stereotest.' *Journal of Paediatric Ophthalmology and Strabismus*, **20**, 72. *(Abstract.)*

Lewis, T., Maurer, D. (1986) 'Preferential looking as a measure of visual resolution in infants and toddlers: a comparison of psychophysical methods.' *Child Development*, **57**, 1062–1075.

MacDonald, M.A., Dobson, V., Sebris, S.L., Baith, L., Vaner, D., Teller, D.Y. (1975) 'The acuity card procedure: a rapid test of infant acuity.' *Investigative Ophthalmology and Visual Sciences*, **26**, 1158–1162.

MacFarlane, A., Harris, P., Barnes, I. (1976) 'Central and peripheral vision in early infancy.' *Journal of Experimental Child Psychology*, **21**, 532–538.

Medical Research Council (1989) *Annual Report 1988/89.* London: MRC.

Miranda, S.B. (1970) 'Visual abilities and pattern preferences of premature infants and fullterm neonates.' *Journal of Experimental Child Psychology*, **10**, 189–205.

Mohn, G., Van Hof-van Duin, J. (1986) 'Development of the binocular and monocular visual fields of human infants during the first year of life.' *Clinical Vision Science*, **1**, 51–64.

28

—— —— Fetter, W.P.F., De Groot, L., Hage, M. (1988) 'Acuity assessment in non-verbal infants and children: clinical experience with the acuity-card procedure.' *Developmental Medicine and Child Neurology*, **30**, 232–244.

Mountcastle, V.B. (1978) 'Brain mechanisms for directed attention.' *Journal of the Royal Society of Medicine*, **71**, 14–28.

Okuda, F.C., Apt, L., Wanter, B.S. (1977) 'Evaluation of the TNO random dot stereogram.' *American Orthoptic Journal*, **34**, 124–131.

Posner, M.I., Rothbart, M.K. (1990) 'The attention system of the human brain.' *Annual Review of Neuroscience*, **13**, 25–42.

Royal National Institute for the Blind (1990) *New Directions: Towards a Better Future for Multihandicapped Visually Impaired Children and Young People.* London: RNIB.

Saye, A., Frisby, J.P. (1975) 'The role of monocularity: conspicuous features in facilitating stereopsis from random dot stereograms.' *Perception*, **4**, 159–171.

Schiller, P.H. (1985) 'A model for the generation of visually guided saccadic eye movements.' *In:* Rose, D., Dobson, V.G. (Eds) *Models of the Visual Cortex.* Chichester: John Wiley, pp. 62–70.

Sheridan, M.D. (1970) 'New appliances: Sheridan–Gardiner test for visual acuity.' *British Medical Journal*, **1**, 108–109.

—— (1976) *Manual for the STYCAR Vision Tests.* Slough: NFER.

Smith, J., Atkinson, J., Braddick, O.J., Wattam-Bell, J., Moore, A.T., Anker, S. (1989) 'Stereopsis, visual acuity and optokinetic nystagmus in strabismic infants before and after corrective surgery: implications for the critical period.' *Ophthalmic and Physiological Optics*, **9**, 466. *(Abstract.)*

Sokol, S., Jones, K. (1979) 'Implicit time of pattern evoked potentials in infants: an index of maturation of spatial vision.' *Vision Research*, **19**, 747–755.

SPORU (1991) *The Scottish Low Birthweight Study.* Glasgow: University of Glasgow Social Paediatric and Obstetric Research Unit.

Teller, D.Y., Morse, R., Borton, R., Regal, D. (1974) 'Visual acuity for vertical and diagonal gratings in human infants.' *Vision Research*, **14**, 1433–1439.

Van Hof-van Duin, J., Mohn, G. (1983) 'Optokinetic and spontaneous nystagmus in children with neurological disorders.' *Behavioural Brain Research*, **10**, 163–177.

—— —— (1984) 'Vision in the preterm infant.' *In:* Prechtl, H.F.R. (Ed.) *Continuity of Neural Functions from Prenatal to Postnatal Life. Clinics in Developmental Medicine No. 94.* London: Spastics International Medical Publications, pp. 93–115.

—— —— (1985) 'The development of visual function in preterm infants.' *Ergebnisse für experimentellen Medizin*, **46**, 350–361.

—— —— (1986a) 'The development of visual acuity in normal fullterm and preterm infants.' *Vision Research*, **26**, 909–916.

—— —— (1986b) 'Visual field measurements, optokinetic nystagmus and the visual threatening response: normal and abnormal development.' *Documenta Ophthalmologica*, **45**, 305–316.

—— —— (1987) 'Early detection of visual impairments.' *In:* Galjaard, H., Prechtl, H.F.R., Velickovic, M. (Eds) *Early Detection and Management of Cerebral Palsy.* Dordrecht, The Netherlands: Martinus Nijhof, pp. 79–100.

—— Pott, J.W.R. (1990) 'A comparison of recognition and grating acuity in normal and very low birthweight children at 5 years of age.' *Investigative Ophthalmology and Visual Science*, **31**, 186. *(Abstract.)*

—— Mohn, G., Fetter, W.P.F., Mettau, J.W., Baerts, W. (1983) 'Preferential looking acuity in preterm infants.' *Behavioural Brain Research*, **10**, 47–51.

—— Evenhuis-van Leunen, A., Mohn, G., Baerts, W., Fetter, W.P.F. (1989) 'Effects of very low birth weight (VLBW) on visual development during the first year after term.' *Early Human Development*, **20**, 255–266.

Walraven, J. (1975) 'Amblyopic screening with random-dot stereograms.' *American Journal of Ophthalmology*, **80**, 893–899.

Wattam-Bell, J., Braddick, O.J., Atkinson, J., Day, J. (1987) 'Measures of infant binocularity in a group at risk for strabismus.' *Clinical Vision Science*, **1**, 327–336.

3
OPHTHALMOLOGY OF VISUAL IMPAIRMENT

William V. Good

This chapter explores two aspects of pediatric ophthalmology: (1) the assessment of children with low vision, and (2) the diseases that affect the visual pathways in children. It is hoped that this overview will provide the reader with an understanding of the ophthalmologic conditions that cause low vision in children.

Pathologic conditions that cause low vision can be separated into those which affect the anterior visual pathways (eyes, optic nerves, chiasm) and those which affect the geniculostriate (posterior) pathways. Each has unique attributes and physical findings (Table 3.1). Distinguishing the site of disease is not simply academic, since treatment may be quite different for each location.

Disorders affecting the anterior visual pathways
Children with uniocular vision loss are usually not visually handicapped. The exception is the occasional child who, as a result of early onset unilateral vision loss, develops monocular nystagmus (Good *et al.* 1993). On occasion, nystagmus 'spreads' to the uninvolved eye, which can degrade visual acuity. Diminished vision is the direct result of the nystagmus, quite contrary to the usual situation in which nystagmus occurs as a result of afferent eye disease.

In this section discussion is limited to disorders affecting both eyes.

General retinal disorders
LEBER'S CONGENITAL AMAUROSIS
One of the most severe congenital retinal disorders is Leber's amaurosis. This is an autosomal recessive condition that causes widespread dysfunction of cone and rod photoreceptor cells. Afflicted children show poor vision under all conditions (*i.e.* dark and light). Visual acuity is seldom better than an ability to appreciate hand motions. Lambert *et al.* (1989) have described a small group of children with retinal dystrophy similar to that of Leber's amaurosis, plus apraxia of eye movements, neonatal breathing abnormalities, and surprisingly good visual acuity (20/50 to 20/100) (Joubert syndrome). However, these children certainly are exceptional in their good vision.

Children with Leber's amaurosis will often demonstrate a normal retinal examination. However, macular colobomata (Moore *et al.* 1985) and optic disc abnormalities (Flynn and Cullen 1975) will occasionally be present. Over time,

TABLE 3.1

Visual findings in conditions affecting the anterior visual pathways and in those affecting the geniculostriate (anterior) pathways

	Visual acuity	Pupil reactivity	Visual fields	Eye movements	Fundus exam
Anterior visual pathways	Diminished	Sluggish; may have afferent pupil defect or paradoxical pupil reaction	Central scotomata	Nystagmus if vision loss at early age	Abnormal, depending on cause
Posterior pathways	Diminished or normal, often variable	Normal	Field loss	No nystagmus	Usually normal

pigmentary alterations of the retina usually occur. For reasons that are unclear, the vast majority of children with Leber's amaurosis have a hyperopic refractive error (Foxman *et al.* 1983). Eye poking becomes a prominent symptom as children reach 4 to 5 months of age (Franceschetti 1947). Later on, cataract and keratoconus, presumably related to eye poking, can develop. Despite all these changes, the level of vision usually remains stable.

Health care providers should be aware that Leber's disease may occur with other systemic abnormalities. Renal disorders (Senior *et al.* 1961), cardiac anomalies (Russell-Eggitt *et al.* 1989), and CNS defects (specifically hypoplasia of the cerebellum) (Nickel and Hoyt 1982) have all been described.

Development in children with Leber's amaurosis is debated. Several authors have warned that such children have significant delays and defects, including the development of symptoms of infantile autism (Rogers and Newhart-Larson 1989). Others have emphasized that they need not do poorly (Nickel and Hoyt 1982).

ACHROMATOPSIA

Achromatopsia is a disorder of the cone population of photoreceptor cells. Rod cells are unaffected. Children will often show a characteristic fast frequency, small amplitude, binocular nystagmus (Yee *et al.* 1981). Indeed, this may be the only form of nystagmus in the first year of life that can be used to diagnose a specific disorder of vision. Additionally, achromats will show photophobia with an onset at approximately 1 year of age, and visual functioning that is far better in the dark than in the light. Visual acuity is usually 20/200 to 20/400. A paradoxical pupil reaction may be present (pupils initially constrict in the dark).

Achromatopsia, also termed rod monochromatism, is usually inherited as an autosomal recessive trait. Clinicians should be aware that occasional children with neuronal ceroid lipofuscinosis will demonstrate a disorder of cone cells as a premonitory sign of more generalized and widespread neurologic disease (Spalton *et al.* 1980).

CONGENITAL STATIONARY NIGHT BLINDNESS (CSNB)

In CSNB, children do not see well in the dark, but see much better under lighted circumstances. In the X-linked variety, boys have nystagmus within the first three months of life and low vision. Female carriers of X-linked recessive CSNB may occasionally show signs and symptoms (Ruttum *et al.* 1992). Children with autosomal recessive CSNB may also develop nystagmus as a result of vision loss. In the autosomal dominant variety, nyctalopia (night blindness) is prominent, but visual acuity under lighted circumstances is relatively preserved.

Almost all children with this disorder have myopia. The electroretinogram (ERG) will typically show markedly diminished scotopic responses, often with a normal A wave, with nearly normal photopic responses. In the X-linked variety, photopic responses to the ERG are also abnormal.

OGUCHI'S DISEASE

Oguchi's disease is a type of stationary night blindness. Inheritance is autosomal recessive. Patients present with nyctalopia (night blindness) and have a green discoloration of the retina under photopic (lighted) conditions. In the dark, the retina appears normal (Mizuo phenomenon).

FUNDUS ALBIPUNCTATUS

In fundus albipunctatus, another type of stationary night blindness, white spots are present in the retina (Krill 1977). Nyctalopia is a prominent symptom.

RETINOPATHY OF PREMATURITY (ROP)

ROP is a disorder of vascularization of the retina. In normal development retinal vascularization proceeds centripetally, from the optic nerve peripherally. The nasal retina is completely vascularized before the temporal retina. The process is completed by 32 to 34 weeks of gestation. Babies born before this time are at risk for arrested vascularization and pathologic neovascularization. When severe, neovascularization can cause scarring and retinal folds or detachment.

The exact cause or causes of ROP are unknown. Infants at highest risk are those with the lowest birthweight. Approximately 50 to 70 per cent of children <1000g, and 90 to 100 per cent of those <500g, will develop ROP if they survive (Bandstra *et al.* 1990). Other risk factors for ROP include gestational age, exposure to light, exposure to increased quantities of oxygen (Campbell 1951), hypoxia, low bilirubin levels, sepsis, and blood transfusions (Aranda *et al.* 1975). Generally, the sicker the baby, the greater the risk of ROP.

Retinopathy is categorized according to the area of the retina involved, and the degree of involvement (Patz 1984). Zone I refers to posterior disease, affecting a full 360° of retina, within twice the distance of the optic nerve to the macula. Zone II disease occurs outside of Zone I, still involving 360°. Zone III disease occurs only in the temporal part of the retina: recall that this is the last area to become vascularized.

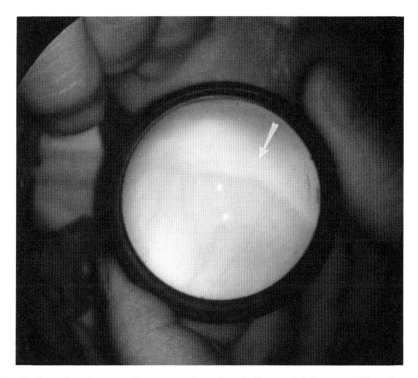

Fig. 3.1. Retinopathy of prematurity, as seen through an indirect ophthalmoscope. Note demarcation ridge (*arrow*) separating vascularized from non-vascularized retina. This baby had stage III ROP.

The severity of ROP is designated by a four stage system. Stage I indicates a demarcation line between vascularized and non-vascularized retina. In stage II the demarcation line becomes elevated. In stage III obvious neovascularization occurs at the demarcation line (Fig. 3.1). Stage IV indicates a subtotal retinal detachment.

Plus disease in ROP indicates shunting of blood between the arterial and venous connections. Dilatation and tortuosity of the blood vessels in posterior aspects of the retina are characteristic, and signify severe disease (Committee for Classification of ROP 1984, Cryotherapy for ROP Co-operative Group 1988). The presence of marked 'plus' disease (see Table 16.11, p. 196) is usually an indication for cryosurgical intervention.

Children with cicatricial retinopathy may be totally blind, and as a result appear to suffer consequences similar to children with other causes of blindness, with important exceptions. The risk of other neurologic disorder in children with blindness from ROP is high. Thus, these children may also suffer cerebral palsy, hydrocephalus and delayed development. Children with bilateral blinding ROP will poke at their eyes. Whether there are actual developmental differences in children with blindness due to ROP (as compared with other causes of blindness) is debated.

ALBINISM

The term albinism encompasses those conditions in which decreased skin and/or eye pigmentation occurs. Children may show light skin pigmentation (tyrosinase positive and tyrosinase negative albinism); some children show an albinotic ophthalmologic examination without cutaneous signs (ocular albinism).

Albinism causes macular hypoplasia (O'Donnell 1984), resulting in mild optic nerve hypoplasia. Most children with albinism show nystagmus as a result of bilateral decreased vision. High refractive errors and strabismus are quite common in children with albinism, and warrant careful follow-up and attention. The iris shows transillumination defects, and the fundus is lightly pigmented.

Albinism can occur in association with two important systemic syndromes. In Hermansky–Pudlak syndrome, a bleeding diathesis occurs in association with pulmonary fibrosis (Summers *et al.* 1988). In Chédiak–Higashi syndrome, slate-gray pigmentation occurs with nystagmus and defects in neutrophils (Bedoya *et al.* 1969); affected children are extremely prone to recurrent infectious diseases.

OTHER DISORDERS CAUSING RETINAL DISEASE

Several neurodegenerative conditions can result in bilateral retinal disease. It is beyond the scope of this chapter to review these in detail. Clinicians should be aware that children with *neuronal ceroid lipofuscinosis* can present with decreased vision. Eventually such children show seizures and hypotonia with intellectual deterioration and death. *Peroxisomal disorders* such as infantile Refsum's disease, Zellweger syndrome and neonatal adrenoleukodystrophy can also cause retinal degeneration in association with neurologic deterioration (Lambert 1991).

A host of conditions lead to blindness from retinal disease associated with sensorineural hearing loss. Usher syndrome (retinitis pigmentosa plus congenital sensorineural hearing loss) is the most common, but many other diseases are known to affect vision and hearing, including infectious diseases (*e.g.* syphilis, rubella) and neurodegenerative diseases (mitochondrial cytopathy, peroxisomal disorders).

Diseases of the optic nerve

OPTIC NERVE HYPOPLASIA

Optic nerve hypoplasia is emerging as a leading cause of low vision in young children. Typically the condition occurs sporadically, with rare cases transmitted in an autosomal recessive fashion. Risk factors include young maternal age, maternal diabetes, and prenatal maternal abuse of alcohol (Stromland 1985), cocaine (Good *et al.* 1992*b*) and hallucinogens (Chan *et al.* 1978). Optic nerve hypoplasia may occur in conjunction with pituitary abnormalities and midline CNS defects (de Morsier 1956).

The diagnosis is based on low vision with or without nystagmus and an ophthalmologic examination that demonstrates small optic nerves. The appearance of the optic nerve may be deceptive. A double ring sign can be mistaken as a

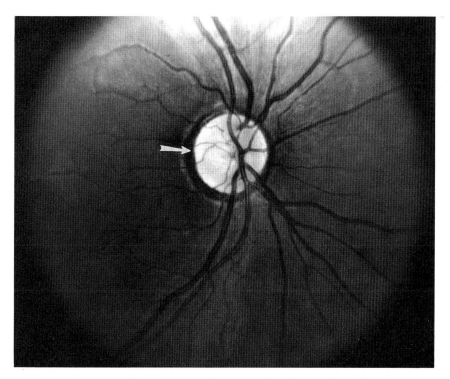

Fig. 3.2. Optic nerve atrophy: note pale optic nerve *(arrow)*.

normal sized optic nerve. In most cases, however, the diagnosis is not in doubt.

Once diagnosed, children with optic nerve hypoplasia should undergo a careful endocrine and neurologic evaluation. Rare cases of optic nerve hypoplasia are caused by congenital tumors of the visual pathways (Taylor 1982). For that reason most should undergo neuroradiologic studies.

OPTIC NERVE ATROPHY

Optic nerve atrophy (Fig. 3.2) causes degeneration of the optic nerves with loss of the nerve fiber layer and pallor of the optic nerve head. Repka and Miller (1988) have reviewed their practice and provided some epidemiologic data as to various causes. Tumors of the visual pathways are probably the most important and frequent cause of optic atrophy. Optic nerve gliomas and craniopharyngiomas are notorious for causing loss of vision due to optic atrophy in one or both eyes. Occasional children demonstrate monocular nystagmus. When the atrophy is severe and bilateral in the first year of life, though, bilateral pendular nystagmus is the rule.

Perinatal hypoxia–ischemia is another cause of optic atrophy, although it is far more likely to cause cortical visual impairment (Lambert *et al.* 1987). Infectious diseases can be etiologic. Certain demyelinating and white matter diseases can also lead to optic atrophy. Autosomal dominant optic atrophy causes bilaterally reduced vision (20/25 to 20/200).

The investigation of the child with optic atrophy should always include neuroradiologic studies. Treatment is directed at the cause of the atrophy.

Congenital cataracts
Advances in microsurgical techniques for treatment of congenital cataracts have led to a greatly reduced incidence of blindness from this cause. Congenital cataracts are usually hereditary or sporadic. Nevertheless, a large number of metabolic conditions and syndromes can cause cataracts (Hoyt and Good 1991). In general, an evaluation of the child with congenital cataracts should be limited to a careful genetic history, unless the child has signs or symptoms of other organ involvement and/or neurologic dysfunction and/or developmental delay.

Prompt treatment of monocular and binocular cataracts can lead to good visual fixation with surprisingly good visual results (Gelbart *et al.* 1982). After surgery for the cataract, the child is rendered aphakic in the operated eye or eyes. Rehabilitation involves various combinations of patching, contact lenses and/or spectacles. Intraocular lenses in young children are debated: most pediatric ophthalmologists prefer not to use them until children are older.

Congenital corneal anomalies
The congenitally opaque cornea offers one of the most important and challenging diagnostic dilemmas for the pediatrician and ophthalmologist (Good and Hoyt 1990). With bilateral opacities, the differential diagnosis includes congenital infections, rubella, glaucoma, exposure keratitis, cystinosis, metabolic diseases of the cornea (particularly mucopolysaccharidoses), scleral cornea, and rare dystrophies of the cornea such as congenital hereditary endothelial dystrophy.

The evaluation of the congenitally cloudy cornea should prompt any effort possible at treatment. In cases of congenital glaucoma, prompt alleviation of the elevated pressure can often be accomplished with surgery, which in turn results in improvement in the cloudiness. Nevertheless, bilateral opacification will frequently lead to the development of nystagmus.

The treatment team is faced with a dilemma with unilateral corneal opacification. The child will usually have good vision in the fellow eye. Treatment is often surgical; unfortunately the time for rehabilitation with unilateral penetrating keratoplasty is so long that some degree of unilateral form deprivation amblyopia occurs. Furthermore, surgical results in the management of unilateral corneal opacities in children have not been nearly so good as they are with management of similar problems in adults.

Ocular colobomata
Ocular colobomata occur when the eye wall fails to completely fuse during

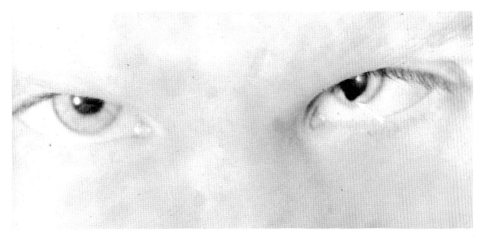

Fig. 3.3. Iris colobomata in a child with CHARGE syndrome (see Table 3.2). Note inferonasal, 'keyhole' iris defect of the left eye.

TABLE 3.2

Conditions which cause optic colobomata

Autosomal dominant: no other systemic abnormalities
CHARGE syndrome (*c*oloboma, *h*eart defect, choanal *a*tresia, *r*etardation, *g*enitourinary defects, *e*ar anomalies)
Goltz focal dermal hypoplasia
Meckel–Gruber syndrome
Lenz microphthalmia syndrome
Trisomy 13
Aicardi syndrome
Peters Plus syndrome

gestation. A cleft or gap in retina and/or choroid and/or iris occurs inferonasally, unilaterally or bilaterally (Fig. 3.3).

The usual cause is autosomal dominant inheritance, but a host of neurologic and genetic conditions can also be etiologic (Table 3.2). When both maculae are involved, nystagmus and reduced vision result.

Cortical visual impairment

Cortical visual impairment (CVI) is a term that has supplanted cortical blindness in describing children with visual abnormalities caused by lesions in the posterior visual pathways (Fig. 3.4). The usual etiology is perinatal hypoxia–ischemia

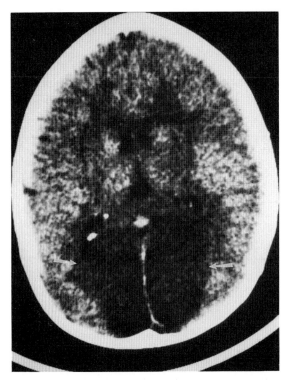

Fig. 3.4. Cortical visual impairment caused by bilateral occipital infarcts (*arrows*).

(Flodmark *et al.* 1990). Congenital infections (meningitis, encephalitis), congenital cerebral defects and hydrocephalus are also relatively frequent causes. The etiology can usually be determined on the basis of physical findings, a careful history and a neuroimaging study.

Physical findings in CVI include normal pupil responses and a normal anterior segment and fundus examination. Usually, no optic nerve atrophy or hypoplasia is found. The retina is normal. The child with CVI may exhibit a constellation of behaviors which help to localize the cause of vision impairment to the posterior visual pathways (Jan and Wong 1991). When vision is quantifiable, it may be variable. The ability to discriminate colorful objects is perhaps better than the ability to see black and white contrasted objects. The peripheral visual fields may be preserved, as these are located in the more anterior aspects of the visual cortex. Because of this, children with CVI will turn their heads and attempt to spot objects of interest with their side vision.

Neuroimaging studies may be extremely valuable in diagnosing CVI. Periventricular leukomalacia, hydrocephalus and watershed infarcts are usually easily examined by CT or MRI. Rarely, the MRI scan will be normal.

The visual prognosis in CVI is debated. Wong (1991) has expressed concern that it is usually poor, but most authorities favor a guardedly optimistic view. When periventricular leukomalacia occurs, the prognosis may be worse than with more posterior (cortical) lesions (Lambert *et al.* 1987).

Delayed visual maturation
There is nothing more disconcerting than the child who has a normal ophthalmologic examination, and perhaps even a normal MRI scan and yet does not show any visual attentiveness. Such children pose an important diagnostic challenge to pediatricians and opthalmologists alike. The term for this condition, when it occurs in the first several months of life, is delayed visual maturation (DVM).

DVM has been classified according to types (Fielder *et al.* 1985). In type I there is no ocular or CNS defect; in type II the delay in visual maturation accompanies neurologic abnormalities; type III occurs in children with infantile nystagmus and albinism; and type IV occurs in the setting of other severe structural eye anomalies.

Fielder *et al.* (1991) reported that congenital anterior visual abnormalities will cause a delay in the normal maturation of vision. Personal experience agrees with this: in the Department of Ophthalmology at the University of California, San Francisco, we have frequently seen children with lesions such as optic nerve hypoplasia with no apparent vision in the first few months of life, who return at age 18 to 24 months showing surprisingly good visual fixation and responses.

Children with DVM invariably improve. Some may be left with residual neurologic abnormalities and for this reason should be followed regularly by a pediatrician with expertise in early child development (Fielder and Mayer 1991).

Amblyopia
Amblyopia is defined as vision loss due to inadequate visual stimulation. The abnormality is located in the visual cortex. As a rule, amblyopia is unilateral and occurs in the absence of any identifiable physical abnormality. However, important exceptions warrant mention.

Bilateral amblyopia can result from bilateral high hypermetropic or astigmatic refractive errors. Treatment of the refractive error will often result in improvement. Unilateral amblyopia can coexist with a pathologic condition, *e.g.* unilateral or asymmetric optic nerve hypoplasia. Patching the better eye will occasionally result in improvement in the amblyopic eye (Kushner 1982).

Visual assessment of children
Primary care physicans will be aware of the difficulties in assessing vision in preverbal or poorly cooperative children. While there is no practical difficulty in measuring visual acuity in an alert and cooperative 8- or 9-year-old, the exact opposite is true for most toddlers. However, visual assessment in very young children is still possible. The health care provider can look for clues to vision from a variety of sources. The following sections discuss (1) visual acuity measurement, (2)

physical findings in children with low vision, (3) behavioral diagnostic aspects of low vision, (4) forced choice preferential looking techniques, (5) optokinetic nystagmus, (6) visual evoked potentials, (7) electroretinography, and (8) visual field examinations. In all categories, the emphasis is on the assessment of children with low vision.

Visual acuity measurement

The gold standard in the ophthalmologic assessment remains the visual acuity examination. Acuity is a function of macular integrity and a measurement of the ability to see a figure of given size at a given distance, *e.g.* a child who recognizes a figure subtending 5″ arc at 20ft (6m) distance is recorded as having 20/20 (6/6) vision. The first number indicates the distance (in feet/metres) between subject and figure; the second number indicates the distance at which the figure subtends 5″ of arc.

Letters and numbers are used to test older children. Illiterate patients can be tested with E's or Landolt broken rings. These tests require that the patient specify the orientation of an E or the gap in a C.

Henry Allen pictures are useful in assessing amblyopia (Mayer and Gross 1990) and some children with bilateral vision loss. The LH symbol test devised by Hyvärinen (1990) can also be quite useful in measuring vision, as it promotes unambiguous, evenly spaced, easily identifiable objects for the child to recognize.

Other aspects of vision should not be ignored (*e.g.* night vision, visual field). Children usually cope with poor acuity far better than adults. Therefore, vision assessment should emphasize how well the child *functions* at home and at school.

Physical findings in children with impaired vision

The alert clinician should look for physical signs of diminished vision in preverbal children. Symmetric and bilateral vision loss in the first year of life, when due to anterior visual pathway disease (*e.g.* retinal dystrophy, bilateral optic nerve hypoplasia), causes nystagmus. This nystagmus may have its onset at any time from birth to several months of age, and its characteristics can be correlated in a rough fashion with a child's actual vision (Jan *et al.* 1986). Slow, pendular nystagmus usually indicates poor vision. Faster frequency, small amplitude nystagmus correlates with better visual acuity. Roving eye movements with nystagmus indicate very low vision, far less than 20/400.

Jan *et al.* (1988) demonstrated that nystagmus with the fellow eye occluded will be worse in the eye with the worst vision. They termed this the unequal nystagmus test. Congenital cone dystrophies (achromatopsia) will also typically show a characteristic nystagmus pattern with a very fast frequency, small amplitude wave form (Yee *et al.* 1981). Otherwise nystagmus cannot be used in any helpful fashion diagnostically. Indeed, even upbeating nystagmus has been reported in a variety of diseases of the anterior visual pathways (Good *et al.* 1990).

Unilateral or asymmetric vision loss in the anterior pathways will cause an afferent pupil defect. Here the pupil on the side of the more pronounced lesion will react less briskly than the fellow pupil. By swinging a flashlight from one eye to the other, the examiner will notice that the pupil in the more normal eye reacts faster to light, and the afflicted eye's pupil reacts less briskly and indeed may even dilate in response to a light that is transferred in front of it (Marcus Gunn pupillary sign).

The paradoxical pupil occurs regularly in achromatopsia and congenital stationary night blindness. Rather than dilating in response to darkness, paradoxical pupils initially constrict (Barricks *et al.* 1977).

Strabismus can occur in children with unequal vision. The usual pattern of deviation is esotropia in the eye with lesser acuity. Presumably an unequal visual input from the two eyes leads to a sensory deficit that allows one eye to deviate from normal alignment. Any child with strabismus should have a careful examination to check whether vision is equal in both eyes.

The refractive error of children can be quite helpful in sorting out eye abnormalities. Myopia in the first year of life is unusual and should suggest the possibility of a congenital retinal disorder or, less likely, ROP. Conversely, severe hyperopia is seen consistently in Leber's congenital amaurosis (Foxman *et al.* 1983).

Another important physical finding that would indicate a cause of visual failure in children is leukokoria. This suggests congenital cataract, retinal infection or retinoblastoma. The ophthalmologist can ascertain the exact cause.

Amblyopia is diagnosed when vision in one eye is abnormal and the physical examination is normal. Since amblyopia can coexist with pathologic conditions, it should be suspected in an eye that is constantly eso- or exotropic, or anisometropic.

Behavioral signs of low vision
Jan and his colleagues should be credited with much of the research in the area of neurobehavioral signs of vision impairment in young children. These signs can be a great benefit in diagnosing vision loss. Their use requires only observational skills on the part of the examiner (Table 3.3).

As mentioned previously, nystagmus in the first year of life will usually indicate bilateral anterior visual pathway disease. Occasionally the nystagmus is difficult to discern. Many children with nystagmus will take a head turn to dampen the nystagmus. The head turn allows a child to find a so-called 'null' position which often is eccentric from the primary position of gaze.

Children with low vision of any cause will hold objects of interest close to their eyes. Nystagmus can be diminished by convergence, with resulting improved vision. Linear magnification also results and causes objects to appear larger.

Eye poking or pressing occurs in children with bilateral retinal disease (Jan *et al.* 1983). Conditions such as cicatricial ROP, hereditary retinal dystrophies and congenital retinal infections will lead to this symptom. Eye poking is a very specific finding and is not found in other causes of vision failure in children. The presumed etiology is that eye poking causes pressure on retinal ganglia cells and allows a sort

TABLE 3.3

Neurobehavioral signs of vision impairment in young children

Location of lesion	Behavioral response
Retina (bilateral)	Eye poking
Anterior pathways (bilateral)	Nystagmus → head turn
Oculomotor control center	Head thrusting
Cortical	Staring at lights Photophobia Use of side vision to pick up objects Preference for colored objects Good navigational skills Variable acuity

of visual stimulation that would not be provided by even the most intense light source. Eye pressing may be responsible for periocular fat atrophy and a sunken socket appearance in children.

A tendency to gaze above objects of interest may occur in children with bilateral central scotomata (Good *et al.* 1992*a*). Examples of diseases that could cause this include bilateral colobomata affecting the macula, and bilateral central scotomata as might occur with certain cases of optic atrophy or toxic optic neuropathies.

Upgaze can occur in other conditions. Occasional children who are otherwise healthy will exhibit tonic upgaze in infancy (Ahn *et al.* 1989). In this situation, upgaze is not a sign of vision abnormality, but rather is a transient supranuclear eye movement disorder that resolves with time.

Hemianopic children turn their heads to the side of the hemianopia but then rotate their eyes back to confront the visual target directly (Good 1991). The purpose of this adaptation is unknown, since the movement of the eyes back toward central fixation would apparently eliminate any adaptation to the head turn. On the other hand, this neurobehavioral sign is seen so consistently with hemianopias that it is of diagnostic importance. Many hemianopic children also develop an exotropia. While we cannot say that this is an actual adaptation, the exotropia does potentially enlarge and expand the visual fields.

Cortical visual impairment can cause a constellation of neurobehavioral signs and adaptations (Jan *et al.* 1987). Light gazing is a pronounced symptom (Jan *et al.* 1990). A preference for colored objects over black and white ones is observed. Children with CVI will also demonstrate variable visual performance. Some show an innate type of 'blind sight' which provides a level of subconscious vision, even in the absence of identifiable objective vision (Schneider 1969). For example, some apparently totally blind children with CVI can ambulate and avoid bumping into objects.

Head thrusting occurs in a condition called ocular motor apraxia (Zee *et al.* 1977). A patient with normal eyes but an inability to move them into a desired field of gaze will thrust her/his head in order to drag the eyes to the desired location. Occasionally the condition is mistaken for blindness in infancy. However, the physical examination is otherwise normal, and the development of head and neck muscle control brings about the diagnostic head thrusting at 4 to 5 months of age.

Forced choice preferential looking
In forced choice preferential looking (FPL), the observer takes advantage of the fact that an infant or young child prefers looking at a patterned stimulus instead of a homogeneous field (Teller 1979). The subject is presented two simultaneous stimuli and her/his visual behavior is observed. If s/he chooses to look at a stimulus with a pattern, this indicates that s/he can see it. If s/he shows no particular visual preference, the observer must interpret either an inability to see the stimulus or poor attention. The size of the pattern stimulus correlates with visual acuity. Drawbacks to this type of vision testing include difficulty interpreting an infant's inattentiveness, and false positives and false negatives. The test is also somewhat labor intensive and requires 10 to 15 minutes to perform, again assuming that the infant is attentive.

FPL has been used to quantify vision in a variety of pathologic conditions. It correlates reasonably well with other methods of assessing vision in CVI (Beril and Bane 1992). FPL can also play a role in assessing delayed visual maturation and other causes of low vision with the following important exceptions. Many visually impaired children suffer abnormalities of eye movement and cannot easily demonstrate the behavioral response necessary for interpretation of FPL. Covering an eye will often degrade vision in the fellow eye in children with nystagmus, because the nystagmus worsens (latent nystagmus).

Optokinetic nystagmus
Optokinetic nystagmus (OKN) is induced when a tape with vertical black stripes is rotated in front of the infant's eye, in a left-to-right or right-to-left arc. It can be used in evaluating children suspected of being blind (Hoyt *et al.* 1982), but most OKN drums and tapes only take up a small portion of the infant's visual field and therefore are subject to false interpretation, *i.e.* the child's vision may be directed above or below them. Some children have difficulty moving their eyes as desired, and this may also be misinterpreted as decreased vision.

Finally, it should be noted that there are two systems involved in creating the OKN response, a subcortical system and a cortical pursuit system. Therefore, children who are cortically blind may demonstrate a reasonably good response, which can be misleading.

Visual evoked potentials
Visual evoked potentials (VEPs) can be administered in two ways. The flash VEP

generates a wave whose amplitude and latency can be used to measure and assess diseases that affect the visual pathways. In particular, demyelinating disease (Regan *et al.* 1976) and compressive lesions of the visual pathways (Halliday *et al.* 1976) can be diagnosed.

Patterned VEPs attempt to measure visual acuity by stimulating the macula. The test usually requires steady gaze fixation, reasonably good attentiveness and good health. Therefore, children with nystagmus, seizures, poor cooperation or ill health are poor candidates for this test (Hoyt 1984). On the other hand, pattern VEP testing is useful in assessing amblyopia, perhaps even under sedation (Wright *et al.* 1986).

My own experience is that VEP testing adds little to the assessment or quantification of low vision in children. False positive and false negative evaluations can be misleading. The clinical examination is most accurate and relevant.

Cortical mapping techniques study larger areas of the brain in a dynamic fashion and are showing promise in the evaluation of children with CVI. In the future, it may be possible to assess CVI more accurately with this technique (Jan and Wong 1991).

Electrophysiology

Electrophysiologic testing is useful in establishing a retinal etiology for vision loss in a young child. The ERG measures the mass response of rod and cone photoreceptor cells. It does not correlate well with actual acuity or visual function and so plays a mainly diagnostic role.

Tests of cone photoreceptor cells are conducted after the patient's eyes have adapted to ambient light; a bright flash then elicits an electrical potential across the retina. In conditions that cause abnormalities of cone photoreceptor cells (*e.g.* achromatopsia), the ERG will be diminished or flattened.

On the other hand, after a prolonged dark adaptation, a low intensity light flash will selectively stimulate rod photoreceptor cells. Congenital stationary night blindness and early onset retinitis pigmentosa are examples of conditions that will cause a diminution of the dark adapted ERG, particularly when compared to the light adapted (photopic) ERG.

Diseases that affect both cones and rods (*e.g.* Leber's congenital amaurosis, retinitis pigmentosa) will cause diminution of response in light and dark adapted testing.

Visual field examinations

The clinician must usually rely on rather indirect evidence in assessing visual field integrity in children, since accurate measurements of integrity require lengthy periods of attention and cooperation. Confrontational testing involves sampling peripheral vision by moving an object in the periphery while the child's gaze is forward. Most children will make a nearly direct saccadic eye movement to the object of interest, if it can be seen. Children who don't see well in a given visual field will usually look past it and then make a corrective eye movement to the target (Zangemeister *et al.* 1982). Hemianopic children will usually turn their heads toward the non-seeing field, and then rotate the eyes back to the object of interest (Good 1991).

Conclusion

The most important aspect of vision assessment is the patient's level of visual functioning in her/his home and school environments. This can only be assessed after careful history taking and a home visit. All other measurements described above should be seen as corroborative; that is, they should lend support and definition to the family's understanding and perception of the child's vision.

REFERENCES

Ahn, J.C., Hoyt, W.F., Hoyt, C.S. (1989) 'Tonic upgaze in infancy: a report of three cases.' *Archives of Ophthalmology*, **107**, 57–58.

Aranda, J.V., Clark, T.E., Maniello, R., Outerbridge, E.W. (1975) 'Blood transfusions: a possible potentiating risk factor in retrolental fibroplasia.' *Pediatric Research*, **9**, 362.

Bandstra, E.S., Bauer, C.R., Onstad, L., Lucey, J.F. (1990) 'Retinopathy of prematurity: prevalence and clinical correlates in very-low-birth-weight (VLBW) infants.' *Pediatric Research*, **27**, 239 (*Abstract.*)

Barricks, M.E., Flynn, J.T., Kushner, B.J. (1977) 'Paradoxical pupillary response in congenital stationary night blindness.' *Archives of Ophthalmology*, **95**, 1800–1804.

Bedoya, V., Grimley, P.H., Dugue, O. (1969) 'Chédiak–Higashi syndrome.' *Archives of Pathology*, **88**, 340–349.

Beril, E., Bane, M. (1992) 'Forced-choice preferential looking acuity of children with cortical visual impairment.' *Developmental Medicine and Child Neurology*, **33**, 722–727.

Campbell, K. (1951) 'Intensive oxygen therapy as a possible cause for retrolental fibroplasia. A clinical approach.' *Medical Journal of Australia*, **2**, 48–50.

Chan, C.C., Fishman, M., Egbert, P.R. (1978) 'Multiple ocular anomalies associated with maternal LSD ingestion.' *Archives of Ophthalmology*, **96**, 282–284.

Committee for Classification of Retinopathy of Prematurity (1984) 'The international classification of retinopathy of prematurity.' *British Journal of Ophthalmology*, **68**, 690–697.

Cryotherapy for Retinopathy of Prematurity Co-operative Group (1988) 'Multicentre trial of cryotherapy for retinopathy of prematurity (preliminary results).' *Archives of Ophthalmology*, **106**, 471–479.

de Morsier, G. (1956) 'Etudes sur les dysraphies cranioencéphaliques. III. Agénéses du septum lucidum avec malformation du tractus optique. La dysplasie septo-optique.' *Schweizer Archiv für Neurologie und Psychiatrie*, **77**, 267–292.

Fielder, A.R., Mayer, D.L. (1991) 'Delayed visual maturation.' *Seminars in Ophthalmology*, **6**, 182–193.

—— Russell-Eggitt, I.R., Dodd, K.L., Mellor, D.H. (1985) 'Delayed visual maturation: ophthalmic and neurodevelopmental aspects.' *Transactions of the Ophthalmological Society of the United Kingdom*, **104**, 653–661.

—— Fulton, A.B., Mayer, D.L. (1991) 'The visual development of infants with severe ocular disorders.' *Ophthalmology*, **98**, 1306–1309.

Flodmark, O., Jan, J.E., Wong, P.K.H. (1990) 'Computed tomography of the brains of children with cortical visual impairment.' *Developmental Medicine and Child Neurology*, **32**, 611–620.

Flynn, J.T., Cullen, R.F. (1975) 'Disc oedema in congenital amaurosis of Leber.' *British Journal of Ophthalmology*, **59**, 497–502.

Foxman, S.G., Wirtschafter, J.D., Letson, R.D. (1983) 'Leber's congenital amaurosis and high hypermetropia: a discreet entity.' *In:* Henkind, P. (Ed.) *ACTA XXIV International Congress Ophthalmology, Vol. 1.* Philadelphia: J.B. Lippincott, pp. 55–58.

Franceschetti, A. (1947) 'Rubéole pendant la grossese et cataracte congénitale chez l'enfant: accompagné du phénomène digitooculaire.' *Ophthalmologica*, **114**, 332–339.

Gelbart, S.S., Hoyt, C.S., Jastrebski, G., Meog, E. (1982) 'Long-term visual results in bilateral congenital cataracts.' *American Journal of Ophthalmology*, **93**, 615–621.

Good, W.V. (1991) 'Behaviors of visually impaired children.' *Seminars in Ophthalmology*, **6**, 158–160.

—— Hoyt, C.S. (1990) 'Corneal abnormalities in childhood.' *In:* Taylor, D.S.I. (Ed.) *Pediatric Ophthalmology*. Oxford: Blackwell Scientific, pp. 178–199.

—— Brodsky, M.C., Hoyt, C.S., Ahn, J.C. (1990) 'Upbeating nystagmus in infants: a sign of anterior visual pathway disease.' *Binocular Vision Quarterly*, **5**, 186–192.

—— Crain, C.S., Quint, R.D., Koch, T.K. (1992a) 'Overlooking: a sign of bilateral central scotomata in children.' *Developmental Medicine and Child Neurology*, **34**, 69–73.

—— Ferriero, D.M., Golabi, M., Kobori, J.A. (1992b) 'Abnormalities of the visual system in infants exposed to cocaine.' *Ophthalmology*, **99**, 341–346.

—— Koch, T.S., Jan, J.E. (1993) 'Monocular nystagmus caused by unilateral anterior visual pathway disease.' *Developmental Medicine and Child Neurology. (In press.)*

Halliday, A.M., Halliday, E., Kriss, A., McDonald, W.I., Mushin, J. (1976) 'The pattern-evoked potential in compression of the anterior visual pathways.' *Brain*, **99**, 357–374.

Hoyt, C.S. (1984) 'The clinical usefulness of the visual evoked response.' *Journal of Pediatric Ophthalmology and Strabismus*, **21**, 231–234.

—— Good, W.V. (1991) 'The eyes.' *In:* Rudolph, A.M. (Ed.) *Rudolph's Pediatrics*. San Mateo, CA: Appleton & Lange, p. 1905.

—— Nickel, B.L., Billson, F.A. (1982) 'Ophthalmological examination of the infant. Developmental aspects.' *Survey of Ophthalmology*, **26**, 177–189.

Hyvärinen, L.H. (1990) *The LH Symbol Tests*. Long Island, NY: Lighthouse.

Jan, J.E., Wong, P.K.H. (1991) 'The child with cortical visual impairment.' *Seminars in Ophthalmology*, **6**, 194–199.

—— Freeman, R.D., McCormick, A.Q., Scott, E.P., Robertson, W.D., Newman, D.E. (1983) 'Eye-pressing by visually impaired children.' *Developmental Medicine and Child Neurology*, **25**, 755–762.

—— Farrell, K., Wong, P.K., McCormick, A.Q. (1986) 'Eye and head movements of visually impaired children.' *Developmental Medicine and Child Neurology*, **28**, 285–293.

—— Greenwald, M., Sykarda, A.M., Hoyt, C.S. (1987) 'Behavioral characteristics of children with permanent cortical visual impairment.' *Developmental Medicine and Child Neurology*, **29**, 571–576.

—— McCormick, A.Q., Hoyt, C.S. (1988) 'The unequal nystagmus test.' *Developmental Medicine and Child Neurology*, **30**, 441–443.

—— Groenveld, M., Sykanda, A.M. (1990) 'Light-gazing by visually impaired children.' *Developmental Medicine and Child Neurology*, **32**, 755–759.

Krill, A.E. (1977) 'Congenital stationary night blindness.' *In:* Krill, A.E. (Ed.) *Hereditary Retinal and Choroidal Disease, Vol. II.* London: Harper & Row, 391–417.

Kushner, B.J. (1984) 'Functional amblyopia associated with abnormalities of the optic nerve.' *Archives of Ophthalmology*, **102**, 683–685.

Lambert, S.R. (1991) 'Degenerative retinal diseases in childhood.' *Seminars in Ophthalmology*, **6**, 219–226.

—— Hoyt, C.S., Jan, J.E., Barkovich, J., Flodmark, O. (1987) 'Visual recovery from hypoxic cortical blindness during childhood.' *Archives of Ophthalmology*, **105**, 1371–1377.

—— Kriss, A., Gresty, M., Benton, S., Taylor, D. (1989) 'Joubert syndrome.' *Archives of Ophthalmology*, **107**, 109–113.

Mayer, D.L., Gross, R.D. (1990) 'Modified Allen pictures to assess amblyopia in young children.' *Ophthalmology*, **97**, 827–832.

Moore, A.T., Taylor, D.S., Harden, A. (1985) 'Bilateral macular dysplasia and congenital retinal dystrophy.' *British Journal of Ophthalmology*, **69**, 691–699.

Nickel, B.L., Hoyt, C.S. (1982) 'Leber's congenital amaurosis: is mental retardation a frequent associated defect?' *Archives of Ophthalmology*, **100**, 1089–1092.

46

O'Donnell, F.E. (1984) 'Congenital ocular hypopigmentation.' *International Ophthalmology Clinics*, **24**, 133–142.

Patz, A. (1984) 'An international classification of retinopathy of prematurity.' *Pediatrics*, **74**, 127–133.

Regan, D., Milner, B.A., Heron, J.R. (1976) 'Delayed visual perception and delayed visual evoked potentials in the spinal form of multiple sclerosis.' *Brain*, **99**, 43–66.

Repka, M.X., Miller, N.R. (1988) 'Optic atrophy in children.' *American Journal of Ophthalmology*, **106**, 191–194.

Rogers, S.J. Newhart-Larson, S. (1989) 'Characteristics of infantile autism in five children with Leber's congenital amaurosis.' *Developmental Medicine and Child Neurology*, **31**, 598–607.

Russell-Eggitt, I., Taylor, D.S.I., Clayton, P.T., Garner, A., Kriss, A., Taylor, J.F.N. (1989) 'Leber's congenital amaurosis—a new syndrome with cardiomyopathy.' *British Journal of Ophthalmology*, **73**, 250–254.

Ruttum, M.S., Lewandowski, M.F., Bateman, J.B. (1992) 'Affected females in X-linked congenital stationary night blindness.' *Ophthalmology*, **99**, 747–752.

Schneider, G.E. (1969) 'Two visual systems. Brain mechanisms for localization and discrimination are dissociated by tectal and cortical lesions.' *Science*, **163**, 895–902.

Senior, B., Friedmann, A.I., Brando, J.L. (1961) 'Juvenile familial nephropathy with tapeto-retinal degeneration.' *American Journal of Ophthalmology*, **52**, 625–633.

Spalton, D.J., Taylor, D.S.I., Sanders, M.D. (1980) 'Juvenile Batten's disease: an ophthalmological assessment of 26 patients.' *British Journal of Ophthalmology*, **64**, 726–732.

Stromland, K. (1985) 'Ocular abnormalities in the fetal alcohol syndrome.' *Acta Ophthalmologica*, Suppl. 171, 1–50.

Summers, C.G., Knoblock, W.H., Witkoop, C.J., King, R.A. (1988) 'Hermansky–Pudlak syndrome: ophthalmic findings.' *Ophthalmology*, **95**, 545–555.

Taylor, D. (1982) 'Congenital tumours of the anterior visual system with dysplasia of the optic discs.' *British Journal of Ophthalmology*, **66**, 455–463.

Teller, D.Y. (1979) 'The forced choice preferential looking procedure: a psychophysical technique for use with human infants.' *Infant Behavior and Development*, **2**, 135–153.

Wong, R.N. (1991) 'Cortical blindness in children: a study of etiology and prognosis.' *Pediatric Neurology*, **7**, 78–185.

Wright, K.W., Eriksen, J., Shors, T.J., Ary, J.P. (1986) 'Recording pattern visual evoked potentials under chloral hydrate sedation.' *Archives of Ophthalmology*, **104**, 718–721.

Yee, R.D., Balch, R.W., Honrubia, V. (1981) 'Eye movement abnormalities in rod monochromacy.' *Ophthalmology*, **88**, 1010–1018.

Zangemeister, W.H., Meienberg, O., Stark, L., Hoyt, W.F. (1982) 'Eye–head coordination of homonymous hemianopia.' *Journal of Neurology*, **226**, 243–254.

Zee, D.S., Yee, R.D., Singer, H.S. (1977) 'Congenital ocular motor apraxia.' *Brain*, **100**, 581–599.

4
NEUROLOGICAL CAUSES AND INVESTIGATIONS

James E. Jan

An endless list of neurological disorders can damage the visual pathways before and after they are fully formed. These include infections, asphyxia, injury, tumours, toxins, increased intracranial pressure, and degenerative, neurological, metabolic and other diseases. The degree of damage and of loss of sight depends on the timing, location, intensity and specificity of the insult. In most instances it is possible clinically to classify visual loss into anterior and posterior visual pathway defects, which at times can coexist. This type of neuroanatomical division is of practical importance, since the neurological signs, visual behaviour and habilitation of children with ocular and cortical loss differ.

In this chapter, the various ocular lesions with neurological causes and the main types of cortical visual impairment (CVI) occurring in children are presented. The routine ocular and neurological examination of visually impaired children will not be discussed, but it will be shown that certain clinical signs, and the understanding of visual behaviours, mannerisms and eye and head movements, are helpful in separating anterior and posterior visual pathway defects.

Neurological causes of anterior pathway defects
Identical ocular and CNS lesions can result from a great number of neurological insults. Thus, optic nerve atrophy can be caused by tumours, inflammation, injury, hereditary and metabolic disorders, and so on (Repka and Miller 1988). Similarly, brain infarcts causing visual loss can be due to injury, vascular disease or increased intracranial pressure. Thus, findings on ophthalmological examination or brain scanning should not be used synonymously with aetiology. Much confusion can be avoided by observing this simple rule.

Visually impaired children with ocular abnormalities frequently have associated medical problems. In one study (Robinson *et al.* 1987), mental retardation was found in 23.0 per cent, cerebral palsy in 18.0 per cent, epilepsy in 13.1 per cent, hearing impairment in 8.2 per cent and heart defects in 14.8 per cent of visually impaired children born in the early 1980s with congenital ocular abnormalities. Over 50 per cent of these subjects had some additional impairment(s). In contrast, all children with CVI have associated neurological problems, which are often numerous and profound. In both groups, further neurological deficits can result from understimulation. These findings clearly demonstrate that many disorders cause simultaneous ocular and brain lesions and that ocular abnormalities can coexist with CVI. Indeed, in a study by Whiting *et al.* (1985), 60 per cent of children with CVI had ocular defects. It has never been shown how many patients with ocular lesions had CVI, but judging from the number of associated neurological disorders, the figure must be substantial. This fact is, of course, very important for those who are involved in the care of these patients.

Blindness can result from ocular and neurological disorders, although the separation is not always clear. For example, in neurocutaneous albinism, visual pathway misrouting is persistently present, thought to be due to the lack of pigmentation (Apkarian 1991). Infants with retinopathy of prematurity (ROP) commonly have associated neurological disabilities. They also sustain far more hypoxic–ischaemic insults during the perinatal period than their normally sighted counterparts, suggesting that there are important neurological factors in the aetiology (Fielder *et al.* 1988, Hoon *et al.* 1988). Children with anophthalmos and microphthalmos frequently demonstrate CNS abnormalities, because development of the brain and the eyes are so closely connected (Warburg 1987).

Longitudinal studies of congenital blindness during the last 30 to 40 years have shown dynamic changes in the prevalence of ocular lesions and their casues, as a result of steady improvements in medical care (Robinson *et al.* 1987). ROP, optic nerve atrophy (ONA) and cataracts are the most common ocular lesions encountered in British Columbia, and the prevalence of all three has decreased. In the mid-'80s the prevalence of ocular 'legal blindness' was 3/10,000 live births, whereas that of acquired ocular 'legal blindness' was only a fifth of that. Unfortunately ROP is again reemerging, due to the survival of extremely low birthweight, low gestational age infants.

The congenital neurological disorders mainly affect the optic nerves, although they can involve every part of the globe. ONA was most frequently the result of asphyxia in term infants, and much less so among those born preterm. These children tended to be severely disabled. There are many other rare causes of congenital ONA, including intrauterine hydrocephalus, tumours, infections, cranial synostosis and cerebral haemorrhage. However, the old-fashioned concept of mechanical injury to the optic nerves during the birth process must be discarded.

In recent years optic nerve hypoplasia (ONH) has become a major cause of blindness. The vast majority of children with ONH demonstrate various endocrine deficiencies and multifocal brain damage, involving more than just the midline structures. Many different neurological insults and CNS anomalies can damage the developing visual pathways and their precursors, thus resulting in ONH (Lambert *et al.* 1987*b*). After the development of the optic nerves is completed, insults produce ONA. It is not an hereditary disorder. In most instances the exact aetiology is unclear. It is most intriguing that this ocular lesion, which during the late '70s and early '80s was a leading cause of blindness, is now becoming less frequent in British Columbia.

Infants with a number of congenital neurological disorders can present with normal or near-normal looking retinas and extinguished electroretinograms. These severely visually impaired children at least initially tend to be diagnosed as having Leber's congenital amaurosis. They must be fully investigated for peroxisomal, mitochondrial and amino acid disorders, infantile lipofuscinosis and Joubert syndrome, among others (Lambert *et al.* 1989*b*). The diagnosis of Leber's amaurosis should probably be restricted to a subgroup of children who have no additional neurological or metabolic problems. Prenatal infections can affect the retina and the brain: toxoplasmosis, varicella, herpes simplex virus, cytomegalo-virus, rubella and others. There are also a few children with developmental abnormalities of the retina who have major CNS malformations (Warburg 1987).

In a study of 97 children with cataracts (Pike *et al.* 1989), causal factors included prenatal infection (35), hereditary cataracts (22), various syndromes and metabolic disorders (9), repeated head trauma (1) and unknown (30). The cataracts were congenital in 90 subjects and acquired in seven. Most of the cases of unknown aetiology represented new mutations of dominantly inherited cataracts. The study showed that preterm birth and associated complications were not a cause of infantile blinding cataracts. Children who were only visually impaired most likely had dominantly inherited cataracts, whereas those with additional disabilities had non-genetic cataracts and needed to be carefully investigated for prenatal infections, metabolic disorders and various syndromes.

There are also a great number of chromosomal defects and syndromes which affect the various structures of the globe and are associated with neurological and somatic abnormalities.

During the 30-year period 1960–1989, only 159 children with acquired ocular blindness have been assessed in our Visually Impaired Program (Robinson and Jan 1993). These children were either born or had been brought to live in British Columbia. They had previously normal sight, which is important to state, because approximately one-third of congenitally visually impaired children later experience deterioration in their sight (Freeman *et al.* 1991).

Optic nerve atrophy, followed by retinal disorders, together constituted more than 90 per cent of acquired ocular lesions with blindness. ONA was caused almost entirely by neurological disorders (Table 4.1), while retinal lesions were mainly genetic in aetiology.

Tumours were the most frequent cause of acquired ONA (38/93): optic nerve gliomas (17), craniopharyngiomas (11) and other intracranial malignancies (10). In the 1980s, optic nerve gliomas continued to occur and resulted in blindness because the loss of vision tended to be gradual, the tumour was relatively symptom-free and treatment was still unsatisfactory. Craniopharyngioma, while now rare, still occasionally leads to blindness.

Injury to the globe and anterior visual pathways was the second most frequent aetiology (35/93) and resulted from different mechanisms. In 18 children ONA was caused by raised intracranial pressure, due to shunt failure (8), late treatment of hydrocephalus (3), astrocytoma (3), chronic subdural haemorrhage (1), Crouzon's

TABLE 4.1

Neurological causes of acquired optic nerve atrophy with legal blindness (N = 93)

Tumours	Optic nerve gliomas	17
	Craniopharyngiomas	11
	Other malignancies	10
Injury	Increased intracranial pressure	18
	Child battering	6
	Firearms	5
	Head traumas	4
	Methyl alcohol	2
Infection and	Encephalitis	3
autoimmune disorder	Meningitis	2
	Uveitis	2
	Optic neuritis	2
	Unknown	5
Heredity	Recessive ONA	3
	Leber's ONA	2
	Neurodegenerative ONA	1

disease (2) or osteopetrosis (1). Child battering resulted in bilateral ONA in six children. Visual loss due to battering was more common, but most of these children also had CVI. The other, rare, causes of injury were firearms, explosives, head injury and methyl alcohol.

Infection, autoimmune and hereditary disorders were the other causes of acquired ONA (Table 4.1).

The neurological causes of acquired blinding retinal disorders were retinoblastoma (11), neurodegenerative diseases (9) and injury (3). Retinoblastomas in the 1980s occurred with possibly the same frequency as before, but because of improved therapy no longer resulted in blindness.

In British Columbia, with a population of around 3 million people, acquired ocular blindness was surprisingly rare during the past 30 years, with an average of about five cases per year. Moreover, the prevalence has now been reduced by two-thirds, mainly because of improved medical care of neurological disorders such as tumours, raised intracranial pressure, infections and certain injuries.

Neurological causes of posterior pathway defects

Permanent CVI has significantly increased in recent years because improved medical care now allows so many critically ill children with severe brain damage to survive. CVI is defined as a temporary or permanent visual loss caused by a disturbance of the posterior visual pathways and/or occipital lobes. While damage to the geniculostriate tracts and visual cortex causes visual loss, lesions of almost any part of the brain can influence visual behaviour. However, children who are visually inattentive or who experience visual–perceptual difficulties but have

TABLE 4.2

Aetiology, CT findings and ocular abnormalities (N = 70)

Aetiology	N	CT findings	Mild optic atrophy
Asphyxia			
Preterm	16	Periventricular leukomalacia	1
Term	17	Diffuse tissue loss; occipital infarcts only (4)	3
Acquired	1	Diffuse tissue loss	1
Malformation	10	Migration defects	2
Trauma	8	Variable pathology	3*
Infection	8	Variable pathology	1*
Shunt failure	6	Bilateral occipital infarcts with dilated lateral ventricles	3
Miscellaneous	4	Diffuse tissue loss (1); unilateral porencephalic cyst (1); normal (2)	1

Adapted by permission from Flodmark *et al.* (1990).
*Two children in these groups also had retinal abnormalities.

normal distance visual acuity, and those with unilateral destruction of the striate cortex causing homonymous hemianopia are not discussed here. 'Cortical blindness', which suggests total loss of sight, is a popular but misleading term, since the majority of children with CVI have some residual vision. Even complete bilateral destruction of the striate cortex does not lead to total absence of sight because of the presence of extrageniculostriate visual pathways (Celesia *et al.* 1980, Campion *et al.* 1983). Therefore the term 'impairment' is more appropriate than 'blindness'.

The study of CVI is still in its infancy. Until recently children with CVI were more or less ignored, and many standard ophthalmology and neurology textbooks do not even discuss this topic.

In a recent study of children with CVI (Flodmark *et al.* 1990), asphyxia was the most common cause (Table 4.2). Due to developmental changes in the vascular anatomy of the brain, ischaemic damage occurs in different locations in preterm and in term infants (Pape and Wigglesworth 1979). In the preterm infant, periventricular leukomalacia due to hypoxic–ischaemic insult can affect both the geniculocalcarine tract and visual cortex (Fig. 4.1). These children commonly have spastic diplegia, but in spite of their severe motor disabilities and CVI are not necessarily mentally retarded. In the term infant, the watershed areas most susceptible to hypoxic–ischaemic injury involve the cortex, including the striate cortex (Flodmark *et al.* 1980). The majority of these children show various degrees of multicystic encephalomalacia on CT scans (Fig. 4.2), and in contrast to the preterm infants they tend to have worse developmental prognoses. In older children, permanent CVI due to hypoxic–ischaemic insult is less common than in preterm and term neonates. The reason for this is not entirely clear. Fewer older children than infants are exposed to hypoxic events, but it is also suggested that

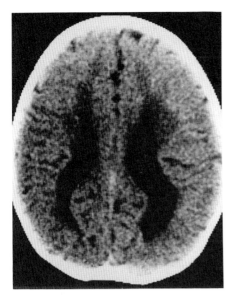

Fig. 4.1. CT scan showing periventricular leuko-malacia. Note the mild ventricular dilatation, the absence of periventricular white matter along the trigonal part of the lateral ventricles, the prominent deep portions of sylvian fissures and the grey matter abutting directly on the lateral ventricles, giving the ventricles an irregular outline. Cortical structures appear normal. (Reproduced by permission from Flodmark *et al.* 1990.)

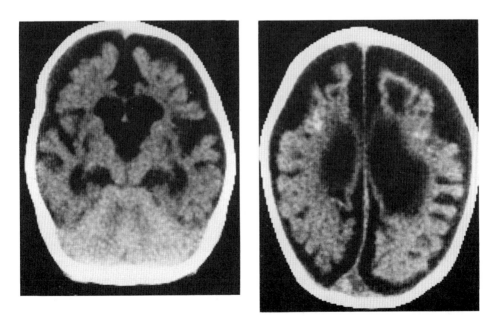

Fig. 4.2. Two CT scans showing multicystic encephalomalacia. Note the dilatation of the ventricular system and the marked loss of cortical grey matter, which is replaced in some areas by cystic spaces. Prominence of subarachnoid spaces over hemispheres and in the interhemispheric fissure is secondary to cortical tissue loss. The head is small. Small dystrophic calcifications are seen as bright spots. (Reproduced by permission from Flodmark *et al.* 1990.)

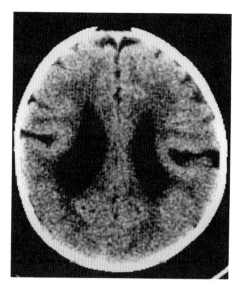

Fig. 4.3. CT scan showing migrational abnormality. Note the mildly dilated lateral ventricles, their dysmorphic shape, and the pachygyria which is a diffuse form of migrational abnormality. The prominent sulci in the parietal lobes represent the 'central sulcus', a primitive structure which is normally replaced by the sylvian fissure as the brain matures. The gyri are broad as the thick cortex is folded in simple patterns throughout the brain. (Reproduced by permission from Flodmark *et al.* 1990.)

with increasing age the visual pathways are more resistant to hypoxic damage (Lambert *et al.* 1987*a*).

Major congenital brain malformations were the second most common cause of CVI (Fig. 4.3). In these children, who tended to be severely multiply disabled, the posterior visual pathways were also affected. In the third largest group, those with trauma, the loss of brain tissue was the direct result of contusions. Depending on the type, severity and area of head injury, the disruption of visual pathways could occur at several levels. Sadly, many of these children are victims of non-accidental injuries. Associated disorders, such as mental retardation, epilepsy, cerebral palsy and other developmental difficulties, are very common in these two groups.

A wide variety of CNS infections can damage the visual pathways at several levels. These will not be discussed here.

Shunt failure in children with hydrocephalus (Fig. 4.4) may produce permanent or temporary CVI (Arroyo *et al.* 1985, Connolly *et al.* 1991). This type of CVI is less common today because of improved neurosurgical care. The most common mechanism is transtentorial herniation, leading to compression of the posterior cerebral arteries against the tentorial edge (Meyer 1920). Infarction of the brain areas supplied by these arteries is likely to happen if the herniation progresses rapidly, because when the process is gradual the developing collateral circulation can limit the ischaemic injury. CT detection of occipital infarcts in children with hydrocephalus and shunt failure provides strong support for the presumed aetiology of transtentorial herniation. Chronically increased intracranial pressure tends to cause optic nerve atrophy.

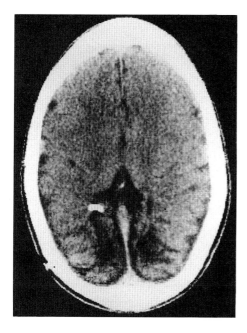

Fig. 4.4. CT scan showing bilateral occipital infarcts. This child with hydrocephalus had an episode of shunt dysfunction during which infarcts developed, involving both posterior cerebral arteries. Note the symmetrical tissue loss in the occipital lobes, the dilated occipital horns and the prominence of subarachnoid spaces over the occipital lobes. Part of the ventricular shunt is seen in the trigone area of the right lateral ventricle. (Reproduced by permission from Flodmark *et al.* 1990.)

Characteristic features of CVI

The behaviour of children with CVI is so characteristic that the diagnosis can be strongly suspected from the history alone. Children with pure CVI do not appear blind. They look with a markedly short visual attention span, but see little, and their visual skills vary from minute to minute. Tiredness, unfamiliar environments, complex visual information, suboptimal lighting, poor contrast, medications, innate processing factors, etc. can all dramatically impede their visual perception. This high degree of visual variability is a common cause of confusion and frustration to the caregivers.

Children, even with severe CVI, are attracted to colours, especially yellow and red, and occasionally are able to name them more easily than objects (Jan *et al.* 1987). This is because colour perception has bilateral hemisphere representation and perhaps because it requires fewer neurons than form perception. Experimental data suggest that the use of colour as a stimulus with forms facilitates the perception of forms by patients with CVI (Merrill and Kewman 1986). This is why teachers who teach these children simple shapes and letters find it helpful to outline them with colour.

About one-third of patients turn their heads to the side in a peculiar fashion when reaching for objects. It is not clear why they do this, but as children with dense homonymous hemianopia turn their heads only to one side, it seems likely that they are using their peripheral visual fields for this function.

One of the most common adaptations to any type of subnormal vision is the close range at which these individuals view objects of interest. The primary gain is magnification. Even in the absence of refractive errors, children with CVI also view objects at close range. Through this mechanism, linear magnification is achieved, but at the same time, by exclusion, complex visual information is reduced to simple units. By this process these children avoid the well-known 'crowding effect', where too much visual input impedes or breaks down visual analysis.

Prolonged, compulsive light gazing is a common feature of CVI, being seen in about 60 per cent of such children (Jan *et al.* 1990). The urge to light gaze can be so intense that some of them gaze into the sun. This, of course, can be dangerous because further visual loss could occur from solar retinopathy. A smaller number of low-functioning light gazers also flicker their fingers in front of their eyes against a light source. This habit appears to be an extension of light gazing. It is not clear why some children with CVI are light gazers and others are not. Patients with pure ocular disorders rarely, if ever, exhibit this behaviour, and when it occurs, as for example in congenital rubella syndrome or ROP, it suggests an associated cortical visual disturbance. Light gazing does not correlate well with the severity of CVI because it is seen even with a mild disturbance of the striate cortex and without significant visual loss. Neither is it related to the cause of CVI. Nevertheless, with recovery from CVI light gazing tends to become less severe, and some children completely outgrow this mannerism.

Photophobia, which is commonly noted in certain ocular disorders, is also observed in association with posterior visual pathway defects. Preliminary studies suggest that about one-third of children with CVI are sensitive to bright light, most minimally, a few severely. In 1976, Denny-Brown and Chambers noted in studies with macaque monkeys that these animals avoided bright lights when both occipital lobes were amputated. The cause of brain insult and the severity of visual impairment do not correlate well, but as children grow the photophobia tends to diminish and may disappear. The pathophysiology of this type of central light sensitivity is not understood.

A few individuals with CVI see only stationery objects. Some have severe tunnel vision, most often due to occipital infarcts (Van Hof-van Duin and Mohn 1984). Patients with ocular disorders and severe peripheral visual field loss also find it difficult to note rapidly approaching visual stimuli. In contrast, some children with occipital lobe damage exhibit a striking ability to detect movement. It has been postulated that in these individuals the temporal crescent (the peripheral part of the temporal field), which is represented at the anterior part of the inferior tip of the calcarine fissure, is preserved. This area is especially sensitive to movement stimuli (Benton *et al.* 1980). The possibility also exists that the ability to detect movement is due to intact extrageniculostriate visual pathways (Celesia *et al.* 1980).

Eye and head movements
The eye movements of visually impaired children can offer important clues about

the onset, type and severity of visual loss (Jan *et al.* 1986). Slowly drifting eye movements, mixed with jerky components, are characteristic of profound and also early onset bilateral ocular visual loss. This kind of roving is not seen in children with pure CVI, whose eye movements tend to be smooth, but with such short visual attention span that they look at things only momentarily.

Sensory nystagmus is the hallmark of anterior visual pathway pathology. It is an instability of fixation caused by congenital or early (before 1 year of age) ocular visual loss, manifested as involuntary, bilateral, predominantly horizontal, rhythmic oscillations with similar amplitude and phase in both eyes, and with complex wave forms. The amplitude and frequency of nystagmus roughly parallel the severity of visual loss. Children whose recognition acuity is better than 20/70 rarely demonstrate visible nystagmus, but as the acuity diminishes, the intensity of the nystagmus increases. Thus, with 20/100 vision in the better eye, the oscillation tends to be rapid and small in amplitude, whereas with 20/400 vision it is slower and wider. Sensory nystagmus is not seen in pure CVI except when there is a coexisting congenital ocular disorder. In this case, when the CVI is mild, the nystagmus is only minimally suppressed, but when it is severe, the nystagmus may even be totally absent.

Many severely brain-damaged children exhibit non-specific tremors and even nystagmus. Similarly, children with CVI, in the absence of ocular defects, can have jerky, abnormal eye movements, together with motor nystagmus. This type of eye oscillation should not be confused with sensory nystagmus.

Children with congenital ocular visual loss tend to have impaired eye movements. Those with distance acuity of 20/100 or better generally shift their gaze smoothly, but when the vision in the better eye is close to 20/200 the eye movements become dyspraxic and begin to be associated with compensatory head movements. When vision is worse, the oculomotor difficulties are also more marked. During pursuit and looking on command, severely visually impaired children move their heads rather than their eyes, and when not actively looking, their heads often hang down. With total absence of sight they cannot voluntarily move their eyes, and these children keep their heads erect only when taught to do so. In contrast, those with late-onset visual impairment retain the smoothness of their eye pursuit, and compensatory head movements are less often observed.

This type of eye movement dyspraxia with compensatory head movements is not seen in children with CVI. However, there is a close relationship between the severity of cortical visual loss and neck control. Children who are sitting propped up, with their heads hanging forward, have very restricted visual environments. This not only impedes the development of their vision but also results in diminished motivation to raise their heads and gain better neck control. In these individuals the periodic use of head-supporting collars appears to help.

During fixation many children with ocular visual loss assume a head tilt with a shift in their gaze. They are using their null zones where the intensity of the nystagmus is least obvious because in this position the involuntary retinal image motion is less and the foveation strategies are better, and so they see slightly better. Children with CVI, especially those with major visual field defects, can also exhibit abnormal head and eye positions and occasionally even eccentric fixation, as do some individuals with macular defects.

Mannerisms

Normal children often display thumb sucking, rocking, head banging, hand flopping and other stereotypic behaviours, which tend to be transient and rarely cause any concern. Visually impaired children can have these and their own specific 'blind mannerisms' such as eye pressing, light gazing, and flicking their fingers in front of their eyes as they stare into lights (Jan *et al.* 1983, 1987).

For the full development of the human brain, including the visual pathways, rich, well-balanced and appropriate environmental stimulation is required. With regard to the visual system, it has been shown in experiments by Kalil (1987) that once kittens' retinal ganglion cells are inactivated with a tetrodotoxin and the action potentials or 'messages' from the eyes are blocked, the maturation of the visual pathways is abruptly arrested. The various types of visual self-stimulation are mediated through the ganglion cells whether the stimulus is pressure on the retina, or light gazing into continuous and/or flashing lights. When there is severe sensory deprivation, the brain creates its own 'self-stimulation', perhaps to ensure the maturation of the neurological systems. This may be an explanation for some mannerisms seen in visually impaired children.

Eye pressing commonly occurs in children with severe ocular visual loss, mainly due to retinal disorders. With variable frequency, duration, strength and individual style, these children press their eyes with the fingers, knuckles, or backs of the hands when they are tired, anxious or bored, and they may even fall asleep with their eyes resting on their fists. This mannerism is not seen in children with total blindness and optic nerve defects, perhaps because in optic nerve lesions the number of functioning ganglion cells and optic nerve fibres is significantly reduced. On very rare occasions severely multiply impaired children with CVI poke their eyes from the side as if 'trying to displace the globe'. The intensity of the pressure can be so marked that the periorbital tissues at times are bruised. Most of these children also have other types of self-abusive behaviour. This mannerism should not be confused with eye pressing.

Visual recovery

Some degree of visual recovery is seen in the majority of children with CVI, while in others it is complete. The improvement tends to be gradual, although occasionally, even after several months of blindness, it is rapid. Parents report that their children begin to react more to their visual environments and are gradually able to see greater distances, start to follow moving objects and reach. The exact mechanism of visual recovery is unclear. Improvements are not limited to younger ages, but can continue several years, even into the teens (Groenendaal and Van

Hof-van Duin 1989). Lambert *et al.* (1987*a*) and Groenendaal *et al.* (1989) summarized the various theories which have been proposed for this. The insult producing the CVI may not cause cellular death but only interruption of protein synthesis of neurons and delay in myelination, dendrite formation and synaptogenesis. Recruitment of adjacent neurons and replacement by supranumerary neurons, rewiring of connections, neurochemical adaptations, collateral axonal sprouting, expansion of the dendritic surface area and the use of extrageniculostriate visual pathways have also been postulated. It is now recognized that the improvement of sight in CVI is a form of delayed visual maturation (Fielder *et al.* 1985, Lambert *et al.* 1989*a*). Frequently these children remain visually inattentive and poor visual learners for years, while psychological tests usually show significant visuomotor perceptual difficulties. Therefore, recovery of acuity cannot be equated with recovery of vision in these children.

Dramatic disappearance of blindness is not seen in children with ocular disorders but improvement is common. In one study, 65 per cent of visually impaired infants were initially diagnosed to be blind, but in later years had partial vision, enough to read print (Jan *et al.* 1986). There are at least three possible reasons for this. The visual acuity of infants is normally severely restricted but rapidly progresses during the first year of life and then slowly continues to improve, even in teenage years (Van Hof-van Duin 1989). As a result, without careful testing, visually impaired children appear to have much worse vision in their infancy. Secondly, some children with ocular visual loss have coexistent CVI from which they may recover. Thirdly, occasionally certain ocular disorders can be associated with delayed visual development, the reasons for which are not clear (Tresidder *et al.* 1990).

Investigations

Visually impaired children require sophisticated and carefully planned investigations on an ambulatory basis, rather than as inpatients. An accurate diagnosis is crucial, not only because they have to live with their visual disabilities for the rest of their lives, but also because without the correct diagnosis it is difficult, if not impossible, to offer prognosis, recurrence rates, counselling and sound advice to the parents and other caregivers. Furthermore, severe visual impairment is a low prevalence disorder and no matter how tragic a diagnosis, we can learn something new from every child.

Visually impaired children frequently have associated medical, educational and psychological problems. The absence of sight makes their upbringing more difficult and more demanding on parents, while the presence of additional disabilities can make the job even harder. It is important, as early as possible after the diagnosis, to evaluate these children in a multidisciplinary fashion and then carefully plan for their habilitation and/or rehabilitation.

Estimation of visual acuity is very difficult in children with CVI, because they tend to be so low functioning and uncooperative. Therefore, Snellen (Recognition) acuity measurements cannot be done in most instances. Clinically it is possible to show them standardized, colourful objects and toys and to observe their visual responses (Whiting *et al.* 1985), but this type of testing tends to be inaccurate. However, preferential looking or grating acuity tests appear to be feasible for preverbal and multiply impaired children (Teller *et al.* 1974, Mohn *et al.* 1988). The use of these is described elsewhere in this book. Preferential looking acuity should not be equated with recognition acuity because they represent different brain functions and can be dramatically different in the same patient with CVI.

If not all, probably the majority of children with CVI have visual field defects. By using kinetic arc perimetry as described by Van Hof-van Duin and Mohn (1984) it is possible to obtain measurements of the size and area of peripheral field loss. Caregivers need to know both the visual acuity and residual field size in order to offer more appropriate care.

The EEG is a valuable diagnostic tool. Jeavons (1964) concluded that the most common EEG pattern in children who were totally blind due to ocular lesions, was similar to that of sighted subjects with their eyes open. The record does not contain posterior slowing or occipital spikes normally, which are signs of occipital lobe disturbance. Those who have more than minimal vision tend to have normally behaving alpha rhythms (Jan and Wong 1988). In contrast, in the majority of children with CVI, the posterior waking background consists of poorly defined, low voltage or invariant activity without an alpha rhythm. However, occasionally children with CVI retain their alpha rhythm. The EEG also often shows multifocal epileptiform activity, especially from the occipital lobes.

The EEG can be used to predict prognosis. Children with normal EEGs are unlikely to develop epilepsy. If they have developmental problems, most likely these will be minor. The presence of normal alpha rhythm, superimposed on normal background, rules out CVI and suggests that the residual vision is at least 'finger-counting' or better. Infants who appear totally blind, but whose EEGs reveal alpha rhythm, will have enough vision later to be print readers (Jan and Wong 1988). Obviously, children with CVI who have mildly abnormal records during their initial assessments tend to have a better chance of visual recovery. On the other hand, a suppressed posterior waking background without alpha rhythm and multifocal epileptiform activity suggests that the neurons in the occipital lobe are substantially reduced in number and do not function normally. Therefore the prognosis for reasonable visual recovery is worse (Robertson *et al.* 1986).

CT or MRI scans are very helpful in understanding ocular lesions (Lloyd *et al.* 1991) and the pathophysiology of CVI (Flodmark *et al.* 1990). These studies can also provide reasonable clues to visual recovery. The extent and location of brain damage is important. Children with CVI associated with severe periventricular leukomalacia, multicystic encephalomalacia, major brain malformation or bilateral brain damage involving the visual cortex or pathways are not likely to recover, even though some visual improvement can be expected in most cases. On the other hand, children with CVI and normal or mildly abnormal CT scans often regain their visual acuity. In other words, both EEG and imaging studies suggest that the greater the damage to the occipital lobes, the less likely is complete recovery. Positron emission tomography studies have drawn similar conclusions (Bosley *et al.* 1987).

In the past, investigators have relied heavily on the use of electroencephalographic visual evoked responses (VERs) to diagnose CVI (Barnet *et al.* 1970, Duchowny *et al.* 1974). Unfortunately their usefulness is limited, and normal flash VER recordings are even occasionally obtained in patients with severe CVI. It is postulated that these normal responses are probably mediated by the extrageniculostriate visual system (Spehlmann *et al.* 1977). More recently, topographical brain mapping techniques have been developed (Duffy *et al.* 1979) and as a result, larger areas of the brain can be studied during visual stimulation in a dynamic manner. Visual evoked potential mapping (VEPM) appears to be more useful than the traditional VER, but only a few major medical centres have access to VEPM studies. As yet, neither VER nor VEPM studies can give a reliable prognosis for visual recovery.

Visually impaired children at times require much more detailed ophthalmological, medical, neurological and genetic tests. The description of these is beyond the scope of this chapter.

Habilitation of children with visual impairment
The problems of these children are often complex and not restricted to vision alone. A multidisciplinary approach is necessary, not just for the diagnosis, but also for the management. Habilitation or rehabilitation is much more than just offering sympathy and a few guidelines from well-meaning individuals. The caregivers must know the numerous scientific principles and need to receive carefully planned training. This topic is discussed elsewhere, but it is important to emphasize that there is a radical difference between the visual habilitation of children with CVI and that of those with ocular visual loss (Groenveld *et al.* 1990).

REFERENCES

Apkarian, P. (1991) 'Albinism.' *In:* Hickenlively, J.R., Arden, G.B. (Eds) *Principles and Practice of Clinical Electrophysiology.* St Louis: Mosby Yearbook, pp. 773–782.
Arroyo, H.A., Jan, J.E., McCormick, A.Q., Farrell, K. (1985) 'Permanent visual loss after shunt malfunction.' *Neurology,* **35,** 25–29.
Barnet, A.B., Manson, J.I., Wilner, E. (1970) 'Acute cerebral blindness in childhood.' *Neurology,* **20,** 1147–1156.
Benton, S., Levy, I., Swash, M. (1980) 'Vision in the temporal crescent in occipital infarction.' *Brain,* **103,** 83–97.
Bosley, T.M., Dann, R., Silver, F.L., Alavi, A., Kushner, M., Chawluk, J.B., Savino, P. J., Sergott, R.C., Shatz, N.J., Reivich, M. (1987) 'Recovery of vision after ischemic lesions: positron emission tomography.' *Annals of Neurology,* **21,** 444–450.
Campion, J., Latlo, R., Smith, Y.M. (1983) 'Is blindsight an effect of scattered light, spared cortex and near-threshold vision?' *Behavioral Science,* **6,** 423–486.
Celesia, G.G., Archer, C.R., Kuroiwa, Y., Goldfader, P.R. (1980) 'Visual function of the

extrageniculo-calcarine system in man. Relationship to blindness.' *Archives of Neurology*, **37**, 704–706.

Connolly, M.B., Jan, J.E., Cochrane, D.D. (1991) 'Rapid recovery from cortical visual impairment following correction of prolonged shunt malfunction in congenital hydrocephalus.' *Archives of Neurology*, **48**, 956–957.

Denny-Brown, D., Chambers, R.A. (1976) 'Physiological aspects of visual perception. I. Functional aspects of visual cortex.' *Archives of Neurology*, **33**, 219–227.

Duchowny, M.S., Weiss, I.P., Heshmatolah, M., Barnet, A. (1974) 'Visual evoked response in childhood cortical blindness after head trauma and menigitis.' *Neurology*, **24**, 933–940.

Duffy, F.H., Burchfiel, J.L., Lombroso, C.T. (1979) 'Brain electrical activity mapping: a new method for extending the clinical utility of EEG and evoked potential data.' *Annals of Neurology*, **5**, 309–321.

Fielder, A.R., Russell-Eggitt, E.R., Dodd, K.L., Mellor, D.H. (1985) 'Delayed visual maturation.' *Transactions of the Ophthalmic Society of the United Kingdom*, **104**, 653–661.

—— Moseley, M.J., Ng, Y.K. (1988) 'The immature visual system and premature birth.' *British Medical Bulletin*, **44**, 1093–1118.

Flodmark, O., Becker, L.E., Harwood-Nash, D.C., Fitzhardinge, P.M., Fitz, C.R., Chuang, S.H. (1980) 'Correlation between computed tomography and autopsy in premature and full-term neonates that have suffered perinatal asphyxia.' *Radiology*, **137**, 93–103.

—— Jan, J.E., Wong, P.K.H. (1990) 'Computed tomography of the brains of children with cortical visual impairment.' *Developmental Medicine and Child Neurology*, **32**, 611–620.

Freeman, R.D., Goetz, E., Richards, D.P., Groenveld, M. (1991) 'Defiers of negative prediction: a 14-year follow-up study of legally blind children' *Journal of Visual Impairment and Blindness*, **85**, 365–370.

Groenendaal, F., Van Hof-van Duin, J. (1989) 'Partial visual recovery in two fullterm infants after perinatal hypoxia.' *Neuropediatrics*, **21**, 76–78.

—— —— Baerts, W., Fetter, W.P.F. (1989) 'Effects of perinatal hypoxia on visual development during the first year of (corrected) age.' *Early Human Development*, **20**, 267–279.

Groenveld, M., Jan, J.E., Leader, P. (1990) 'Observations on the habilitation of children with cortical visual impairment.' *Journal of Visual Impairment and Blindness*, **84**, 11–15.

Hoon, A.H., Jan, J.E., Whitfield, M.F., McCormick, A.Q., Richards, D.P., Robinson, G.C. (1988) 'Changing pattern of retinopathy of prematurity: a 37 year clinical experience.' *Pediatrics*, **82**, 344–349.

Jan, J.E., Wong, P.K. (1988) 'Behaviour of the alpha rhythm in electroencephalograms of visually impaired children.' *Developmental Medicine and Child Neurology*, **30**, 444–450.

—— Freeman, R.D., McCormick, A.Q., Scott, E.P., Robertson, W.D., Newman, D.E. (1983) 'Eye-pressing by visually impaired children.'- *Developmental Medicine and Child Neurology*, **25**, 755–762.

—— Farrell, K., Wong, P.K., McCormick, A.Q. (1986) 'Eye and head movements of visually impaired children.' *Developmental Medicine and Child Neurology*, **28**, 285–293.

—— Groenveld, M., Sykanda, A.M., Hoyt, C.S. (1987) 'Behavioural characteristics of children with permanent cortical visual impairment.' *Development Medicine and Child Neurology*, **32**, 755–759.

—— —— —— (1990) 'Light gazing by visually impaired children.' *Developmental Medicine and Child Neurology*, **32**, 755–759.

Jeavons, P.M. (1964) 'The electro-encephalogram in blind children.' *British Journal of Ophthalmology*, **48**, 83–101.

Kalil, R.E. (1987) 'Synapse formation in the developing brain.' *Scientific American*, **261**, 76–85.

Lambert, S.R., Hoyt, C.S., Jan, J.E., Barkovich, J., Flodmark, O. (1987*a*) 'Visual recovery from hypoxic cortical blindness during childhood. Computed tomographic and magnetic resonance imaging predictors.' *Archives of Ophthalmology*, **105**, 1371–1377.

—— —— Narahara, M.H. (1987*b*) 'Optic nerve hypoplasia.' *Survey of Ophthalmology*, **32**, 1–9.

—— Kriss, A., Taylor, D. (1989*a*) 'Delayed visual maturation. A longitudinal clinical and electro-physiological assessment.' *Ophthalmology*, **96**, 524–529.

—— —— —— Coffey, R., Pembrey, M. (1989*b*) 'Leber's congenital amaurosis: a follow-up and diagnostic reappraisal of 75 patients.' *American Journal of Ophthalmoloy*, **107**, 624–631.

Lloyd, I.C., Demaerel, P., Kendall, B.E., Taylor, D. (1991) 'MRI and CT in pediatric ophthalmology.

62

A guide to their use.' *Seminars in Ophthalmology*, **6**, 169–181.

Merrill, M.K., Kewman, D.G. (1986) 'Training of color and form identification in cortical blindness: a case study.' *Archives of Physical Medicine and Rehabilitation*, **67**, 479–483.

Meyer, A. (1920) 'Herniation of the brain.' *Archives of Neurology and Psychiatry*, **4**, 387–400.

Mohn, G., Van Hof-van Duin, J., Fetter, W.P.F., de Groot, L., Hage, M. (1988) 'Acuity assessment in non-verbal infants and children: clinical experience with acuity card procedure.' *Developmental Medicine and Child Neurology*, **30**, 232–244.

Pape, K.E., Wigglesworth, J.S. (1979) *Haemorrhage, Ischaemia and the Perinatal Brain. Clinics in Developmental Medicine No. 69/70.* London: Spastics International Medical Publications.

Pike, M.G., Jan, J.E., Wong, P.K.H. (1989) 'Neurological and developmental findings in children with cataracts.' *American Journal of Diseases of Children*, **143**, 706–710.

Repka, M.X., Miller, N.R. (1988) 'Optic atrophy in children.' *American Journal of Ophthalmology*, **106**, 191–193.

Robertson, R., Jan, J.E., Wong, P.K. (1986) 'Electro-encephalograms of children with permanent cortical visual impairment.' *Canadian Journal of Neurological Sciences*, **13**, 256–261.

Robinson, G.C., Jan, J.E. (1993) 'Acquired ocular visual impairment in children from 1960–1989.' *American Journal of Diseases of Children*, **147**, 325–328.

—— —— Kinnis, C. (1987) 'Congenital ocular blindness in children.' *American Journal of Diseases of Children*, **141**, 1321–1324.

Spehlmann, R., Gross, R.A., Ho, S.U., Leestma, J.E., Norcross, K.A. (1977) 'Visual evoked potentials and postmortem findings in a case of cortical blindness.' *Annals of Neurology*, **2**, 531–534.

Teller, D.Y., Morse, R., Barton, R., Regal, D. (1974) 'Visual acuity for vertical and diagonal gratings in human infants.' *Vision Research*, **14**, 1433–1439.

Tresidder, J., Fielder, A.R., Nicholson, J. (1990) 'Delayed visual maturation: ophthalmic and neuro-developmental aspects.' *Developmental Medicine and Child Neurology*, **32**, 872–881.

Van Hof-van Duin, J. (1989) 'The development and study of visual acuity.' *Developmental Medicine and Child Neurology*, **31**, 543–552.

—— Mohn, G. (1984) 'Visual defects in children after cerebral hypoxia.' *Behavioural Brain Research*, **14**, 147–155.

Warburg, M. (1987) 'Ocular malformations and lissencephaly.' *European Journal of Pediatrics*, **146**, 450–452.

Whiting, S., Jan, J.E., Wong, P.K.H., Flodmark, O., Farrell, K., McCormick, A.Q. (1985) 'Permanent cortical visual impairment in children.' *Developmental Medicine and Child Neurology*, **27**, 730–739.

5

EFFECTS OF VISUAL DISABILITY ON BEHAVIOUR AND THE FAMILY

Maryke Groenveld

It may be hard to believe, but children behave to a large extent the way we expect them to. In every society there are certain behavioural requirements of children at a given age. Children learn to adjust by testing their behaviour against these expectations and observing the reactions of those around them. Their behaviour is shaped by how they 'see' the environment and how the environment sees them.

When a child is visually impaired, the process of adapting to society will differ from that of normally sighted children. Social clues which rely on vision to be understood (*e.g.* body language) may be only partially, or not at all accessible. Understanding of cause and effect, and the relationships between people and/or objects, may differ because of limited or absent visual input (Davidson and Nesker Simmons 1984, Groenveld 1990). In addition, society itself may have different expectations of visually impaired people than it does of the normally sighted, and therefore present them with a different model (Kekelis and Andersen 1984). For instance, if society expects visually impaired people to be helpless, this increases their chances of becoming so, regardless of the circumstances.

Fortunately, societal expectations are not static. A greater awareness of the specific problems and needs of visually impaired children will make society's behavioural model more accessible to them and thus enable them to become better integrated adults.

Over the past 20 years, the population of visually impaired children has changed considerably (Robinson *et al.* 1987). Additional neurological problems are much more common, and the needs of children with cortical visual impairment (CVI) are now recognized as being different from those of children with an ocular impairment (Jan *et al.* 1987, Groenveld *et al.* 1990). Furthermore, in many areas the cultural make-up of the population, its inherent expectations of behaviour and its perception of the disability have become much more diverse (Waxler-Morrison *et al.* 1990). 'Clean' studies about the interaction of cultural/environmental factors, type and degree of visual impairment and additional neurological factors are hard to come by, or even impossible to do, considering the low incidence of visual impairment. However, there are felt to be some commonalities in the circumstances and the behaviour of visually impaired children which warrant further attention.

Diagnosis

The vast majority of cases of visual impairment in children are congenital or perinatal in nature (Robinson *et al.* 1987). This means that by and large the diagnosis is made very early in life. The immediate reaction in many of the parents is shock and disbelief, which not infrequently turns into dislike of the person imparting the news, usually the ophthalmologist. It can lead to feelings of guilt and depression, as well as fear of not being able to take appropriate care of the visually impaired child. However, a lot of the fear of the unknown is shared by first-time parents of typical children, who may not necessarily voice it. Sometimes it may be difficult to discriminate between the effects of post-partum depression and depression with regard to the disability.

Since so many of the impairments are hereditary, it is important that genetic counselling is made available to the parents. However, availability of such a service does not necessarily mean a decrease in incidence of the particular condition. In the case of parents with a genetic visual impairment themselves, not to have children for this reason would constitute a denial of the value of their own lives. For parents who are fully sighted, the desire for a normally sighted child, if the visually impaired child is the first born, can be more overwhelming than the statistical information. Furthermore, not all parents fully understand that the risk factor applies to every single pregnancy, rather than the total number.

In their need to know, parents often press the physicians into predictions about future development. This can be very risky. In our clinic, the number of parents who have said with great contempt 'When he was born the doctor said he was going to be a vegetable, and look at him now' is about balanced by those who have stated 'The doctor said he was going to be fine and not to worry, but I always knew there was something wrong.' In both cases the confidence in physicians can be seriously affected. In infants there may be further brain damage which is not yet evident, or the appropriate tests have not yet been done. Occasionally the child who initially has seemingly very bleak prospects may show a fair degree of spontaneous recovery. This is especially the case with certain groups of children with CVI (Robinson *et al.* 1987). Since the large majority of children with CVI have additional impairments (Groenveld *et al.* 1990) it is important that the parents understand that the visual attentiveness may improve, but not the associated conditions.

Multicultural issues

Twenty-five years ago, the patient population at our clinic was much more homogeneous than it is now. Since it is virtually impossible to interpret behaviour separately from the cultural context in which it occurs, it is important that the professionals involved in evaluations and recommendations familiarize themselves as much as possible with the culture-bound perceptions and expectations of the people they encounter. For example, in some clinics it is customary to address the appointment letter to the parents and confirm the appointment schedule with the mother. This implies that the mother will accompany the child to the assessments. However, in some cultures it is the mother-in-law who has most authority in child-rearing practices.

Even such 'neutral' issues as developmental milestones can be affected by cultural expectations (Hopkins and Westra 1989). If cultural parameters are ignored and the behaviour is only interpreted in the clinician's own frame of reference, the intervention may become very unproductive; converserly, when cultural factors are assumed to play a predominant role, the nature of the behaviour may not be analysed further.

Case history

An 8-year-old Chinese boy was referred to our clinic because of a significant visual impairment. His teacher reported that he was fine academically, but that he was so over-indulged by his Chinese-speaking grandmother who took care of him while his parents worked, that he was very rude and ill-disciplined at school, which interfered with his general achievement. The mother had been told on several occasions that she had to change her child-rearing practices if she wanted her son to succeed in school. She found this very difficult, because at home her mother-in-law was in charge. A detailed investigation revealed, however, that this boy had, in addition to his visual impairment, a significant problem with language processing, which went beyond having English as a second language. His behaviour was entirely appropriate in circumstances where he knew what was required of him.

Issues of grieving, guilt, status in the extended family, etc. may differ considerably from one culture to the next (Waxler-Morrison *et al.* 1990). These factors have a significant effect on the family's interpretation of professional advice and their ability to follow it.

Hospitalization

Since about 50 per cent of children with an ocular impairment (Robinson *et al.* 1987) and almost all of the CVI children (Groenveld *et al.* 1990) have additional disabilities, it is not surprising that visually impaired children often have prolonged stays in hospital early in life. This reduces considerably the opportunities for contact and communication between the new parents and their child and makes it more difficult for them to gain confidence in their parenting abilities. For severely-to-totally visually impaired children these early separations are all the more difficult, since for them early learning depends almost entirely on tactile information. Some hospitals recognize this and foster as much handling by the staff and the parents as the infant can comfortably deal with. There is, however, a delicate balance, since an infant with multiple impairments can easily be over-stimulated and may react with agitation or withdrawal.

Early intervention

The complex needs of a visually impaired child, with or without associated impairments, usually lead to a change in lifestyle for the family from birth onwards. Initially there may be frequent doctor and/or hospital visits. Once the child's condition is diagnosed, support services may be involved, which often entails visits to clinics or visits from profesisonals to the home. Although there is no doubt that these interventions are beneficial (Sonksen *et al.* 1991), especially for skill development, they may also make it more difficult for the parents to develop a natural, responsive parenting style, and they may tend to trust 'expert' advice more than their own observations and intuitions. Occasionally, if visits are spaced far apart, the parents may continue to implement suggestions beyond their periods of usefulness.

Involvement of a number of professionals who do not have contact with each other can result in an assortment of exercise and treatment strategies with little awareness of overlap, or sometimes even seemingly conflicting advice. Multi-disciplinary assessments, where the professionals involved in the evaluation meet with each other and with the families to try to achieve an integrated intervention programme, can reduce the confusion to some degree (Jan and Robinson 1989). Sometimes the parents take care of this problem themselves, such as the mother who commented when she was handed yet another sheet of 'useful' information, 'Oh, this is for my box.' When she was asked what she meant, she said: 'I have a box in my basement for all the papers you people give me. That way I know where they are when people ask and I don't have to read them.'

Family relationships

The arrival of a child with a disability affects the entire family profoundly. Expectations of the child and family life in general have to be adjusted, and the financial burden, even in countries with nationalized health care, is considerable (Query *et al.* 1990, Worley *et al.* 1991). In developed countries, the majority of mothers now go out to work, most out of economic necessity. For families with a disabled child it may be very difficult for both parents to work, or to achieve the same career goals as typical families (Baldwin *et al.* 1983).

In spite of all the stresses a disabled child places on family relationships (Bicknell 1983), there is no clear evidence of a higher incidence of marital dissolution (Hirst 1991). This does not mean, however, that the quality of the marriage is unaffected. In our clinic some parents have stated that they felt it brought them closer together, while others seem to experience the contrary. Kokkonen *et al.* (1991) did find a greater divorce rate among parents of disabled children, when these children were interviewed in adulthood. This may imply that some parents are so involved in the care of their disabled children when they are still living at home, that they do not evaluate their own relationships to the point of taking action, or feel that they cannot in the light of the circumstances. This hypothesis requires further investigation. In the author's personal experience, it is felt that a large amount of the emotional energy of the parents is invested in the disabled child. Problems between the parents are often felt to be minor in comparison and thus are not dealt with when the children are still young. Frequently, one parent becomes more and more focused on the disabled child, while the other tends to be more peripherally involved. Both parents may experience a feeling of isolation, which they perceive as unavoidable, but which may be alleviated through sufficient respite care and/or parental support groups. Even in cases where respite care is available, feelings of guilt or anxiety may prevent the parents from making full use of it. Parents often need help to accept help.

Siblings

Since the visually impaired population is very diverse in its make-up, and visual impairment is a low incidence condition with a large number of possible associated problems, it is difficult to find studies which lend themselves to general statements about siblings. It is undeniable that the presence of a visually impaired child in the family has an effect on the siblings, and vice versa, but predicting the nature of this effect is far more difficult. Parental, as well as societal attitudes toward people with disabilities will influence the attitude of the siblings as well. Contrary to popular belief, living with a disabled child does not always result in a greater understanding of the disability (Steinzor 1967). Jan *et al.* (1977) reported an incidence for behaviour problems of about 26 per cent among the siblings of visually impaired children, but did not describe the nature or severity of these problems. They pointed out that the experiences of siblings of visually impaired children are different from those of typical siblings, because they are less free to express resentment and they may have to adopt a protective role early on. This tendency to involve siblings in adult roles is also expressed by Powell and Ahrenhold Ogle (1985), who in their book about siblings of disabled children devote a relatively small section to the effect of the disability on the siblings themselves. The major emphasis is on how to train siblings as teachers of the disabled child. Although siblings undeniably can have an important role in the habilitation of a disabled child (Weinrot 1974, Craft *et al.* 1990), not much is known about the effects of this kind of systematic involvement on the siblings themselves and what the long term consequences are of encouraging them to assume a parental/teaching role at an early age. Putting a sibling in a teaching role for a large part of the time may also not be entirely a blessing for the visually impaired child, who already lives in a much more intervention oriented climate. Learning to share, participate, support, etc. are not skills which lend themselves well to direct teaching. They are acquired more readily in an environment where children, visually impaired or otherwise, have an equal call on their parent's and each other's love and attention and are faced with some degree of benign competition.

The tolerance of siblings of disabled children is likely to fluctuate with age. In the young adolescent period, when it is very important for children to conform, they may be more embarrassed by having a sibling who is 'different' than they are at other ages. In fact, this is the age where many children are embarrassed to have any siblings or other relatives at all. The nature of the intervention, either by parents, support groups or professionals, will have to take the needs of the siblings themselves at their particular age into consideration. Parents may need some assistance in knowing how, and how much, they can explain about the visual impairment to the siblings at different ages.

The presence of associated problems may also affect the family's ability to cope or the sibling's level of tolerance and support. When the siblings are younger than the visually impaired child, especially if there are other disabling conditions, they may find it difficult to understand that certain behaviours are expected of them but are not expected of their older brother or sister. They may see this as unfair favouritism and may try to get their parents' attention or approval in other ways. This can sometimes result in behaviour problems, which on the surface bear no relationship to the visual impairment of the sibling, but which may be indirectly related (Jan *et al.* 1977).

Adaptive versus deviant behaviour
As stated earlier, the behaviour of visually impaired children is shaped by an alteration in the perception of their environment, due to their visual limitations, in addition to the factors which affect typical children. Their behaviour, therefore, may reflect an adaptation to the different information they receive, rather than a deviation. On the surface it may be difficult to see the difference (Groenveld 1990). Several studies have reported a high incidence of psychiatric disorder in blind children (Cruickshank 1964, Jan *et al.* 1977). However, since the criteria for this type of diagnosis are based on a sighted population and therefore imply access to visual information, it is initially difficult to tell if one is dealing with the outward symptoms of a psychiatric disorder, or the disorder itself. This would not be a problem if in both cases the treatment of choice would be the same, but often it is not. It is very important, therefore, that the diagnosis regarding behavioural deviance is made by a psychiatrist thoroughly familiar with visually impaired and blind children.

It is interesting to note that Freeman *et al.* (1991) found in a 14-year follow-up study of legally blind children, that the diagnosed incidence of psychiatric disorder at the mean age of 22 years, although substantial (32 per cent), was lower than it had been when they were children (57 per cent). It should be pointed out that mental retardation is considered a psychiatric disorder under the DSM-III-R classification (APA 1987), and that multiply disabled individuals were included in this study.

Autistic features in the behaviour of totally blind children are quite common. Stereotypic movements, such as flicking hands or fingers, rocking, spinning, body swaying, twirling, tapping, etc. are seen in blind children (Jan *et al.* 1977) as well as autistic children (Howlin and Rutter 1987). Problems with social interaction and communication are frequently present in both groups, but may result from different causes. Relationships between autism and retinopathy of prematurity need to be treated with caution as well (Keeler 1958, Chase 1972), since it may be difficult to determine to what degree complications resulting from the prematurity play a role. Rogers and Newhart-Larson (1989) reported a relationship between autism and Leber's congenital amaurosis, but this study involved only five children with Leber's disease and would need further validation. Certainly, in our clinic we have seen a number of children with Leber's disease who did not display any autistic features.

Mannerisms such as eye pressing and prolonged light gazing seem to be more common only in the visually impaired group. Eye pressing appears to be most frequent in children with a retinal disorder (Jan et al. 1983), while light gazing would seem to be an indication of CVI (Jan et al. 1991).

Rather than labelling the sterotypic behaviour of blind children as autistic, it may be more productive to see to what degree it can be modified. It can be an expression of under-stimulation, in which case providing an activity which is meaningful to the child may stop it. In some cases, self-stimulative behaviour can indicate over-stimulation. This is especially common in children with CVI, who tend to withdraw into repetitive behaviours when their environment is visually too complex to deal with (Groenveld et al. 1990). If children are able to behave more 'appropriately' once their environment has been made perceptually more accessible to them, the behaviour is more likely a result of the visual impairment, rather than an underlying personality disorder.

In assessments, behaviour check-lists can provide information about what is going on, but the interpretation of the results should be made with the specific circumstances of the child in mind and preferably by someone who is familiar with visually impaired children (Groenveld 1990).

Conversely, equal care should be taken that the behaviour is not automatically attributed to the visual impairment when it may be due to something else. Visually impaired children can have additional learning disabilities, emotional problems or language disorders which are compounded by the impairment but not the direct result of it.

Case history

A 15-year-old girl was referred to the clinic with a moderate visual impairment. She was cutting classes and experimenting with sexual relationships and drugs. She frequently referred to her visual problems and stated that she would rather be known as a drug addict than as visually impaired. She was bright and physically attractive. Her impairment was not directly noticeable to an outsider, nor did it appear to cause her any significant problems in school. She had access to the appropriate support services. Further investigation revealed a long-standing conflict with her mother as well as other family problems, which were unrelated to the visual impairment.

Living in a dysfunctional family, abuse and neglect may affect severely visually impaired children more seriously than typical children, because of their greater dependency.

Modification of mannerisms

Most young, profoundly visually impaired children seem to enjoy some form of self-stimulating activity. They generally tend to be less active than typical children because they are not visually attracted to stimulation around them. Since the developing brain does want input, they frequently turn to their own body as a source of activity (Scott *et al.* 1985).

Unfortunately, understanding the origins of a particular kind of behaviour is not enough to break the habit. Excessive rocking, swaying, hand flapping and other motor mannerisms may suggest that more motor activity is required. Introduction of more vigorous exercise may be of considerable help. Limiting activities to places where it is appropriate may make the habit less noticeable (rocking in a rocking chair or on a rocking horse only, for instance). Giving children something interesting to play with when they are inactive may help reduce the need for stereotypic behaviour. Verbal cueing may be needed to alert children to the fact that they are eye pressing or rocking. Some children prefer the use of a codeword to remind them, rather than always being told not to.

Enrolment in a programme where there are other children around may also help in reducing mannerisms. In our clinic we have noticed that with the tendency toward full integration of visually impaired children in the school system, some mannerisms are not seen as frequently as before, especially among the higher functioning children. It is felt that the accompanying change in peer pressure is to a large extent responsible (Jan and Groenveld 1993).

Body language

The interpretation of behaviour and body language is to a large extent dependent on the previous experience and expectations of the observer. Congenitally totally blind children are not aware of the body language of others, nor of the reaction of others to their own, unless they are specifically taught. Partially sighted children, who may have to make some behavioural adaptations to make their sight more functional, may unknowingly communicate body language which implies feelings they are not necessarily experiencing. This can lead to a number of misunderstandings.

Case history

A 16-year-old boy with a macular disorder and eccentric fixation was referred to the clinic with a history of lack of motivation and a sullen attitude. Indeed, during the assessment he stared over the head of the examiner and his face was rather expressionless. When asked where he was looking, he stated, 'At your face.' He was then asked to lower his eyes until he made eye contact from the examiner's point of view. When she asked where he was looking now, he blushed and said, 'At your chest.' He was advised to do so occasionally during a social conversation.

Although children who have to rely on their peripheral vision cannot and should not always make eye contact, it is socially important for them to do so occasionally.

Similarly, totally blind children should be taught to turn their heads to the listener. However, children who adopt a head tilt to achieve the nystagmus null-point should not be advised by their teachers to 'sit up straight', since this does not serve any social purpose and will interfere with optimal vision.

Language

One of the most common misconceptions about blind children is that they are equally or more adept in language skills than their normally sighted peers (Burlingham 1961, Fraiberg 1977). However, most of the earlier work in this field tended to use instruments which relied heavily on auditory memory skills, rather than comprehension. More recent studies found that language of visually impaired children was more self-oriented and that the word meanings were more limited for them than for normally sighted children (Andersen et al. 1984, Kekelis and Andersen 1984). This was felt to be not only because they missed visual references, but also because far less integrated information was provided for them by their parents.

A higher incidence of echolalia, both immediate and delayed, is reported for blind children (Burlingham 1972), which is possibly an expression of better developed auditory memory skills in blind children, in addition to a lack of information through other senses. There appears to be support in the literature that visually impaired children are more aware of the presence of auditory clues in conversations than are their normally sighted peers (Blau 1964, Flichten et al. 1991), but this does not guarantee the correct interpretation of the implied correct meaning (Blau 1964, Minter et al. 1991). Especially in congenitally blind children, verbal reasoning skills seem to lag behind auditory memory skills (Groenveld and Jan 1992). This can lead to a rather stilted use of language, especially in social situations, where children have to adapt to quickly changing topics, or incorporate broader meanings of words.

Cognitive development

Not only language development is affected by the visual impairment, but the whole process of cognition. The experiences of severely visually impaired children are not the same as those of the fully sighted. Vision enables us to perceive objects in their totality and in relationship to their surroundings. Severely visually impaired children have to rely on sequential observation. They can see or touch only part of an object and have to build up an image from the components. Awareness of the relationships with other objects usually does not occur until much later, and initially the connection between sound and object is often not made. For example, young blind children who are learning to drink from a cup often drop the cup when they are finished because they are unaware of the relationship between the cup and the table. The cup usually appears in mid-air (in the caregiver's hand) and is replaced in mid-air.

For drawing conclusions from sequential information, a higher level of cognitive maturity is needed than for interpreting simultaneous observations. This makes some tasks more difficult to learn for visually impaired children than for normally sighted children of the same age. Sight also provides children with a powerful incentive for learning. They are attracted by all kinds of visual lures and will go and investigate, often to the despair of their parents. Blind babies are in that sense often much better behaved. They tend to be more passive and less inclined to go in search of new experiences. The amount of time they spend per activity in meaningful exploration is usually shorter as well, especially before the establishment of the concept of object permanence (the realization that an object is still there, although it is momentarily hidden from view). Very young normally sighted children know that what they dropped on the floor is still there, because they can see it. They are free to pick it up again, or have it picked up for them, and resume exploration. For a blind child of the same age, the object is gone. Therefore, young severely visually impaired children tend to have fewer learning experiences in the same time period than normally sighted children do. This may slow down their rate of intellectual growth, but not their capacity for it.

Early intervention programmes can be very helpful in providing these children with a greater range of learning experiences, especially the ones which encourage the child to explore more independently.

Social integration
One of the most frequently voiced concerns at our clinic, other than health and academic progress, is the ability of visually impaired children to form lasting relationships with their peers. Parents often describe their children as having a great desire to belong to a group, but not quite knowing how to go about it. In partially sighted children, this wish to be the same as everyone else is sometimes carried to the point of denying the visual impairment altogether. This can lead to difficult and sometimes even dangerous situations. In one instance a young man in his late teens preferred to tell his dates that his driving licence had been revoked due to a drinking and driving conviction, rather than admit to a visual impairment (Freeman *et al.* 1991). In school it can mean that students may refuse to use low vision aids to avoid standing out. Although education about visual impairment and promoting tolerance in the peer group are important, in the period when children shift their focus from family norms to peer group norms, it may be very difficult for adult interveners to break through the patterns.

Teasing/bullying
Not surprisingly, teasing and bullying are reported by parents and children alike as a frequent problem in school. It is not just the visually impaired child who is singled out: all children who are perceived by their peer group as 'different' are potential targets. Some strategies have been developed to help children who are bullied to deal with their attackers more effectively (Ross and Ross 1984, Rosenburg 1985). However, these techniques may require some modification for visually impaired

73

children. Making peers more familiar with the condition through special classroom sessions has frequently been found helpful. In addition to helping the children learn to cope with harassment, strengthening their social skills can also have a beneficial effect. For instance, one of our patients, a 7-year-old girl, is microcephalic, has a retinal disorder and her acuity is 20/200. She is an independent, outgoing girl who is well liked by her peers. When someone at school starts to tease her about her appearance, they find that they not only have to deal with her, but with the rest of her classmates as well.

Academic integration

Full integration in regular schools is becoming more and more the norm, especially on the North American continent. It provides children with a variety of appropriate role models, but it also puts them at risk of not being specifically taught those behaviours which could ease their social integration. Social skills literature is available (Huebner 1986, Swallow and Huebner 1987), but in overcrowded classes and with only limited time available from the itinerant teacher for the visually impaired it is not always feasible to put a social skills training programme in place, especially if the visually impaired child is the only one in the school. Parents can be of invaluable help, maybe not by trying specifically to teach their children how to get on with their peers, but by promoting independence and self-help skills, encouraging an interest in what is going on around them and by introducing hobbies which can be shared by others.

Case histories

Thirteen-year-old Jenny has retinitis pigmentosa. Her central vision is 20/40 but her fields are severely restricted. Her development is delayed and she has severe verbal apraxia. She communicates in a combination of single words, signs and gestures. Formal testing of her cognitive abilities would place her in the moderately retarded range with little scatter. She lives on a farm in a small community. In school she is enrolled in a life skills programme with an aide and partial integration. She is exposed to a lot of practical experiences, both at home and at school. She is encouraged to be as independent as safety allows and, like her siblings, is responsible for specific chores on the farm. She enjoys outdoor activities, especially horseback riding, which she shares with friends of the same age. In spite of her language problems, vision problems and limited general ability, she is a very social child. She contributes actively to social interactions in a very pleasant manner, and people generally enjoy her company. Her friends invite her along on outings, which provides her with the kind of peer experiences adults cannot supply her with.

Dawn, also 13, has bilateral cone dystrophy and a visual acuity of 20/200. Her verbal skills are highly developed, not only those depending on auditory memory skills but also her verbal reasoning skills. Visual perceptual skills are less advanced, partially because of her restricted acuity, but also because of her hesitancy to try anything she is not sure she can excel in. She comes from a somewhat dysfunctional family with a very dominating father who tends to belittle her as well as her mother and brother. Social contacts outside the house are discouraged. Dawn spends most of her time alone. Her communication style is very adult-like, and outside of the classroom she has no peer exposure. Cognitively, her development appears to be much more advanced than emotionally. Over time, she appears to be withdrawing more and more because she has less to share with her peers and she has limited skills in initiating contact. At this point she is doing well academically, although her teachers are concerned about her social isolation.

When Jenny and Dawn are compared, Dawn is much brighter intellectually, but Jenny seems to be much better prepared to meet the challenges of her everyday life. She is learning what her strengths and limitations are and how she can get help when she needs it. Dawn is very skilled in theoretical problem solving strategies, but has very little practical ability. She does not know how to approach her peers and they tend to avoid her. Her family does not see this as problematic and is not providing her with skills and experiences that can be shared. Although for both girls their visual problems are to some degree restricting them, it is not the attribute that determines them.

Academic skills are very important, and visually impaired children need encouragement and support to help them get the education which best enables them to become contributing, independent, fulfilled adults. However, it is often the social skills that determine the quality of day-to-day life, even for the most multiply disabled visually impaired child. The child who will never become independent and will always have to rely on others, will still have to learn how to become a good employer of caregivers. This can mean something as basic as learning to show acknowledgement of the other person. It may require a great deal of time and sensitivity to accomplish this, as well as the support and understanding of the educational authorities.

Summary

The visually impaired child needs to develop, just as normally sighted children do, a healthy self-concept. Since they live in a predominantly sighted world, they have to acquire to the most feasible degree the habits and customs of this world. However, this process should take place in such a way that they do not have to sacrifice their personal identity. Visually impaired children are not children from whom something has been taken away; they have perceptions and experiences which are uniquely their own and which need to be shared and developed. Therefore, in addition to contact with normally sighted people, visually impaired children also need contact with other visually impaired people.

REFERENCES

Andersen, E.D., Dunlea, A., Kekelis, L.S. (1984) 'Blind children's language: resolving some differences.' *Journal of Child Language,* **11**, 45–64.
APA (1987) *Diagnostic and Statistical Manual of Mental Disorders. 3rd Edn—Revised.* Washington, DC: American Psychiatric Association.
Baldwin, S., Godfrey, C., Staden, F. (1983) 'Childhood disablement and family incomes.' *Journal of Epidemiology and Community Health,* **37**, 187–195.

Bicknell, J. (1983) 'The psychopathology of handicap.' *British Journal of Medical Psychology*, **56**, 167–178.

Blau, S. (1964) 'An ear for an eye: sensory compensation and judgement of affect by the blind.' *In:* Davitz, J.R. (Ed.) *The Communication of Emotional Meaning.* New York: McGraw-Hill, pp. 113–127.

Burlingham, D. (1961) 'Some notes on the development of the blind.' *Psychoanalytic Study of the Child*, **16**, 121–145.

—— (1972) *Psychoanalytic Studies of the Sighted and the Blind.* New York: National Universities Press.

Chase, J.B. (1972) *Retrolental Fibroplasia and Autistic Symptomatology.* New York: American Foundation for the Blind.

Craft, M.J., Lakin, J.A., Oppliger, R.A., Clancy, G.M., Van der Linden, D.W. (1990) 'Siblings as change agents for promoting the functional status of children with cerebral palsy.' *Developmental Medicine and Child Neurology*, **32**, 1049–1057.

Cruickshank, W.M. (1964) 'The multiple handicapped child and courageous action.' *International Journal for the Education of the Blind*, **14**, 65–75.

Davidson, I.F.W.K., Nesker Simmons, J. (1984) 'Mediating the environment for young blind children: a conceptualization.' *Journal of Visual Impairment and Blindness*, **78**, 251–255.

Flichten, C.S., Judd, D., Tagalakis, V., Amsel, R., Robillard, K. (1991) 'Communication cues used by people with and without visual impairments in daily conversations and dating.' *Journal of Visual Impairment and Blindness*, **85**, 371–378.

Fraiberg, S. (1977) *Insights from the Blind.* New York: Basic Books.

Freeman, R.D., Goetz, E., Richards, D.P., Groenveld, M. (1991) 'Defiers of negative prediction: a 14-year follow-up study of legally blind children.' *Journal of Visual Impairment and Blindness*, **85**, 365–370.

Groenveld, M. (1990) 'The dilemma of assessing the visually impaired child.' *Developmental Medicine and Child Neurology*, **32**, 1105–1109.

—— Jan, J.E. (1992) 'Intelligence profiles of low vision and blind children.' *Journal of Visual Impairment and Blindness*, **86**, 68–71.

—— —— Leader, P. (1990) 'Observations on the habilitation of children with cortical visual impairment.' *Journal of Visual Impairment and Blindness*, **84**, 11–15.

Hirst, M. (1991) 'Dissolution and reconstitution of families with a disabled young person.' *Developmental Medicine and Child Neurology*, **33**, 1073–1079.

Hopkins, B., Westra, T. (1989) 'Maternal expectations of their infant's development: some cultural differences.' *Developmental Medicine and Child Neurology*, **31**, 384–390.

Howlin, P., Rutter, M. (1987) *Treatment of Autistic Children.* Chichester: Wiley & Sons.

Huebner, K.M. (1986) 'Social skills.' *In:* Scholl, G.T. (Ed.) *Foundations of Education for Blind and Visually Handicapped Children and Youth.* New York: American Foundation for the Blind, pp. 341–362.

Jan, J.E., Groenveld, M. (1993) 'Visual behaviours and behavioural adaptation to visual loss in children.' *Journal of Visual Impairment and Blindness*, **87**, 101–105.

—— Robinson, G.C. (1989) 'A multidisciplinary program for visually impaired children and youth.' *International Ophthalmology Clinics*, **29**, 33–36.

—— Freeman, R.D., Scott, E.P. (1977) *Visual Impairment in Children and Adolescents.* New York: Grune & Stratton.

—— —— McCormick, A.Q., Scott, E.P., Robertson, W.D., Newman, D.E. (1983) 'Eye pressing by visually impaired children.' *Developmental Medicine and Child Neurology*, **25**, 755–762.

—— Groenveld, M., Sykanda, A.M., Hoyt, C.S. (1987) 'Behavioural characteristics of children with cortical visual impairment.' *Developmental Medicine and Child Neurology*, **29**, 571–576.

—— —— —— (1990) 'Light-gazing by visually impaired children.' *Developmental Medicine and Child Neurology*, **32**, 755–759.

Keeler, W.R. (1958) 'Autistic patterns and defective communication in blind children with retrolental fibroplasia.' *In:* Hoch, P.M., Zubin, J. (Eds.) *Psychopathology of Communication.* New York: Grune & Stratton, pp. 64–83.

Kekelis, L.S., Andersen, E.S. (1984) 'Family communication styles and language development.' *Journal of Visual Impairment and Blindness*, **78**, 54–65.

Kokkonen, J., Saukonen, A.L., Timonen, E., Serlo, W., Kinnunen, P. (1991) 'Social outcome of handicapped children as adults.' *Developmental Medicine and Child Neurology*, **33**, 1095–1100.

Minter, M.E., Hobson, R.P., Pring, L. (1991) 'Recognition of vocally expressed emotion by congenitally blind children.' *Journal of Visual Impairment and Blindness*, **85**, 411–415.

Powell, T.H., Ahrenhold Ogle, P. (1985) *Brothers and Sisters, a Special Part of Exceptional Families*. Baltimore: Brookes.

Query, J.M., Reichelt, C., Christoferson, L.A. (1990) 'Living with chronic illness: a retrospective study of patients shunted for hydrocephalus and their families.' *Developmental Medicine and Child Neurology*, **32**, 119–128.

Robertson, R., Jan, J.E., Wong, P.K.H. (1986) 'Electroencephalogram of children with permanent cortical visual impairment.' *Canadian Journal of Neurological Science*, **13**, 256–261.

Robinson, G.C., Jan, J.E., Kinnis, C. (1987) 'Congenital blindness in children 1945–1984.' *American Journal of Diseases of Children*, **141**, 1321–1324.

Rogers, S.J., Newhart-Larson, S. (1989) 'Characteristics of infantile autism in five children with Leber's congenital amaurosis.' *Developmental Medicine and Child Neurology*, **31**, 598–608.

Rosenberg, E. (1985) *Getting Closer*. New York: Berkeley Books.

Ross, D.M., Ross, S.A. (1984) 'Teaching the child with leukemia to cope with teasing.' *Issues in Comprehensive Pediatric Nursing*, **7**, 59–66.

Scott, E.P., Jan, J.E., Freeman, R.D. (1985) *Can't Your Child See? 2nd Edn.* Austin, TX: Pro-ed.

Sonksen, P.M., Petrie, A., Drew, K.J. (1991) 'Promotion of visual development of severely visually impaired babies: evaluation of a developmentally based programme.' *Developmental Medicine and Child Neurology*, **33**, 320–335.

Steinzor, L.V. (1967) 'Siblings of visually handicapped children.' *New Outlook for the Blind*, **61**, 48–52.

Swallow, R.M., Huebner, K.M. (Eds) (1987) *How to Thrive, Not Just Survive*. New York: American Foundation for the Blind.

Warren, D.H. (1984) *Blindness and Early Childhood Development. 2nd Edn.* New York: American Foundation for the Blind.

Waxler-Morrison, N., Anderson, J., Richardson, E. (1990) *Cross-cultural Caring*. Vancouver, BC: University of British Columbia Press.

Weinrot, M.R. (1974) 'A training program in behaviour modification of siblings of the retarded.' *American Journal of Orthopsychiatry*, **44**, 362–375.

Worley, G., Rosenfeld, L.R., Lipscomb, J. (1991) 'Financial counselling for families of children with chronic disabilities.' *Developmental Medicine and Child Neurology*, **33**, 679–689.

6
EFFECT OF SEVERE VISUAL IMPAIRMENT ON DEVELOPMENT

Patricia M. Sonksen

The content of this chapter reflects experience with over 600 severely visually impaired (SVI) babies and preschool children seen since 1977 in the Developmental Vision Clinic at The Wolfson Centre, London. The nucleus of the team for this research/service clinic has been a developmental paediatrician (the present author), a psychologist and a specialist nurse. Most babies have been followed regularly to between 4 and 7 years of age for developmental, visual and paediatric assessment and management; close working partnerships with the departments of Ophthalmology and Genetics at the Hospitals for Sick Children (Great Ormond Street, London) have added substantially to the breadth and depth both of service offered to families and of research perspectives. Visual diagnoses encountered among these patients span the full spectrum of visual and paediatric disorders causing severe degrees of congenital visual impairment in the Western world (see Chapters 1, 3 and 4). One or more major disabilities and/or ongoing disease processes have been found in 60 per cent, and the disorder is genetically determined in approximately 55 per cent.

The simple charm of normal infant development belies its complexity. Observed behaviours reflect the functional integrity of the nervous system, sense organs and musculoskeletal system. Vision is the main input sense for many aspects of development and contributes substantially to most; and because all five senses interact and are to a large degree interdependent, the impact of severe visual impairment on development is wide-ranging and cumulative, especially in the early months.

During the first year, development can be considered in two phases which merge into one another (Sonksen 1983a). The *global* phase spans the first four months, during which awareness of self, parents and surroundings grows, and attributes essential to development, such as drive, interest and communicative interaction, are awakened. The *integrative* phase spans the next eight months and is characterized by sensorimotor and intersensory integration, the formation of basic concepts fundamental to verbal and non-verbal development, and the emergence of motor skills governing speech, manipulation and mobility. All are in jeopardy when a baby is severely visually impaired.

In sighted babies the development of vision—acuity, binocularity, fields and neuromotor ocular functions such as fixation, following, tracking, pursuit, accommodation and convergence—is particularly rapid during the first year (see Chapter 2). Evidence suggests that in children with congenital SVI, full (albeit limited) potential for vision is sometimes never achieved and visual development is often slower than could be achieved with appropriate intervention (Sonksen 1983, Sonksen *et al.* 1991). If levels of vision and visual functioning are suboptimal, developmental progress in other areas is likely to be curtailed.

The global phase
During this phase development is at risk from the impact both upon parents of discovering that their baby is disabled and upon the baby in the process of becoming 'alive' to the world and to her/himself within it.

Parents play a major role in early development; mutual enjoyment of daily experiences and interaction acts as a catalyst for developmental progress. Cultural, social and economic factors influence the range and quality of experience provided by parents, but their emotional state is even more crucial. Shock, sadness, anxiety and depression are natural reactions to news that a baby is disabled, and to the experiences associated with the diagnostic process, identification or exclusion of other disabilities, genetic counselling and early treatment. Alterations in the patterns of responsiveness of such infants add to the stress felt by parents; for example, SVI infants do not return the gaze of their parents, they adopt a passive expression when talked to and, without the forewarning given by sight, may startle and cry when picked up. The resultant emotional exhaustion makes the challenge of parenthood very daunting and diminishes the quality of interaction which is so important to these infants (Sonksen 1989).

Vision provides the sighted infant with a fascinating and dynamic perspective of the world to capture her/his interest and thus arouse a quality of personality which throughout life will fire the mind and body to achieve greater things. Mary Sheridan aptly called this quality *drive*. A parent's eyes and face convey both love and a sense of communication, perfect ingredients for the initiation of emotional and interactive development. When this visual perspective is absent there is a real risk that these essential qualities will remain dormant; experience suggests that if an SVI infant fails to develop interest and responsiveness beyond internal feelings of comfort and discomfort during the first few months of life, they become increasingly difficult to promote.

The early months are therefore critical, and providing parents with experienced emotional support and developmental counselling becomes a priority the moment the diagnosis of SVI is suspected. The diagnosis is frequently made by a specialist—ophthalmologist, paediatrician or paediatric neurologist—working in a regional centre situated some distance from the patient's home: this is appropriate for the provision of specialist medical care and developmental assessment but not for the provision of ongoing emotional support for parents, for which effective liaison between the specialist department and a local team is essential.

In the UK the quality of such services varies from good to non-existent

(McKendrick 1991). At district level the service pool consists of a family health visitor and general practitioner, and the Community Paediatric Service—which may have a 'Vision Team' within its 'Disability Team'. In addition, most Local Education Authorities now provide an advisory or peripatetic teacher of the visually impaired to visit families at home. Ideally, someone in the specialist team (nursing officer, senior orthoptist, social worker) should be responsible for initial, 'on the spot' support at the time of diagnosis and for immediate liaison with the district services. A scheme currently being piloted at the ophthalmology clinic, The Hospitals for Sick Children, may provide a useful model. A specialist health visitor from the Developmental Vision Clinic (DVC) is present while the opthalmologist sees the baby. Afterwards she supports the parents in their distress and attempts to rekindle their joy in the baby and their confidence in themselves as parents. For example, she may explain that the blank expression on the baby's face when they talk to her/him is not disinterest, but the way such babies listen; she will then show how the baby's face comes alive when her/his hands are placed on the parents' faces while they talk. She may arrange an appointment at the DVC and/or show them the illustrated developmental guide (Sonksen and Stiff 1991) we have written for such parents. She will explain how each branch of the local services can help, and that she will personally contact their health visitor, the community paediatric team and the peripatetic advisory teacher after they have left.

The integrative phase

Existence, substantiality, meaning and position in space are attributes of the surroundings normally conveyed mainly through vision to an as yet immobile infant: they form the building-blocks of many cognitive and motor skills. This education process starts at birth, but only crystallizes into demonstrable concepts and skills during the integrative phase. For example, a newborn baby sees, as well as hears, a rattle shaken in front of her/him; s/he possesses an eye- and head-turning reflex to confirm its presence, nature and position when it is shaken beyond her/his field of vision to either side. By 5 months of age the auditory and visual inputs have been integrated and assimilated cortically into an appreciation that sound implies the presence of an object, and cognitive and motor skills have developed to the point where the child can locate the object within an arc at ear level.

The continuing role of vision is evident in the two-stage response of a 7- to 9-month-old to sounds made above and below ear-level: the infant turns and looks to the correct side, but only directs the gaze upwards or downwards once the source impinges upon her/his peripheral vision. The problems faced by an SVI baby in acquiring this skill are obvious, so too are the depth of experience and level of expertise required of clinicians responsible for testing the hearing of such babies —an assessment of paramount importance in those deprived of a major sense.

Other processes influenced by vision during the first year of life (Sonksen 1983b, Sonksen et al. 1984) include: realization of the functional potential of the arms and hands for reaching, grasping and manipulation, and of other parts of the body for mobility; refinement and coordination of movement patterns (locomotor and manipulative); kinaesthetic and tactile sensitivity; stereognosis; localization of touch; emergence of postural and saving reactions; and concepts underlying comprehension of language, cause and effect, spatial relationships, and the structure and composition of the environment.

A developmental model for management
The medical model is discussed in Chapters 7 (ophthalmic) and 8 (paediatric). A developmentalist approaches disability in babies and very young children with a view to designing practical intervention strategies to incorporate into daily routines to counter or circumvent constraints upon development imposed by the disability. Through assessment, a profile of developmental achievement, the nature and severity of impairment, and the constraints imposed by poor vision and by additional impairments upon progress toward the next stage are established for each aspect of development. Strategies are devised by the assessment team which use the sensory inputs and cognitive and motor skills currently available to the baby as advantageously as possible.

Assessment
The Reynell–Zinkin Developmental Scales for Visually Handicapped Children (Reynell 1979) explore five areas of cognitive understanding: social adaptation, sensorimotor understanding, language (comprehension and expression), and exploration of the environment. The sequence within each scale is valuable in identifying those skills which need to be consolidated further and the next one to aim for; they also permit comparison between children with similar degrees of visual impairment. Methods for assessment of hearing and hearing behaviours, and of fine and gross neuromotor development (including postural and saving mechanisms), require considerable adaptation from those used for sighted children.

Planning guidance
Babies learn from daily experiences and interactions within their family; SVI babies are no exception, and care needs to be taken that developmental strategies designed for them are natural rather than contrived. Sighted 1-year-olds enter their second year with basic skills and understanding, ready and eager to refine both. In contrast, their SVI peers are likely to be far less well equipped, with a great deal still to learn about 'how they work and how the world works'.

To illustrate this point we can take the example of the impact of SVI on the development of sound-localizing skill in three 8-month-old boys. A Nuffield high-frequency rattle shaken at ear level half a metre to one side is unlikely to elicit a turn of the head nor any visible change in facial expression or general behaviour. On the other hand, the splash of milk in a bottle (discovered from discussion with the mother to be a source of interest) induces stillness and a listening expression in baby A, an eager expression but no head turn or reaching movement in baby B, and an eager expression and a tentative reach forwards in baby C. Each baby demonstrates a different combination of the areas of understanding required for location of sound: Baby C (i) is familiar with the sound, (ii) relates it to his bottle, (iii) appreciates that the bottle is present, (iv) realizes the potential of his upper limbs for reaching, but cannot (v) accurately locate the sound; Baby B demonstrates (i) and (ii) and not (iii), (iv) or (v); while Baby A shows only (i). Effectively, those concepts not understood are *constraints* operating for that baby. In the design of intervention each constraint is separately addressed. Assume for the moment that all three babies are totally blind. The mother of baby C could be advised to guide the baby's hand to familiar sound sources situated anywhere in a plane horizontal with his ears, coupled with an explanation of why moving the source into his hand might confuse the learning process. Baby B needs strategies to develop awareness of his hands for reaching and concepts of permanence; the bottle and familiar noise-making toys should be used. Before deciding on the starting point of guidance for baby A, further assessment is needed to establish whether or not he shows (ii), (iii) or (iv) in relation to his mother's voice when she leans over and talks to him.

Although the response pattern of each baby to a familiar sound has been demonstrated, their hearing has not been adequately assessed; all three responses indicate that a splash of milk was heard. The peak decibel level of this broad band sound can be gauged with a sound level meter, but the assessor should also attempt to engender the baby's interest in a standard test instrument, such as the Nuffield rattle, by placing it in his hand and helping him to shake it. If interest is gained, the rattle becomes a valid test tool. Personal experience suggests that the optimal test distance for distraction tests in SVI babies is the baby's arm's length, because relatively louder sounds made further away induce a less clear-cut or apparently no behavioural response. Again, the level of sound reaching the ear can be checked with a sound level meter.

Early visual assessment
Vision contributes in such a major way to so many aspects of development that it is logical to use any available/residual vision maximally in each child's developmental programme, and to ensure that visual development is up to full potential at all times. To achieve this, in-depth visual assessment is required, embodying medical or functional approaches.

The first priority when SVI is suspected in a baby is examination at a specialist eye clinic. Ophthalmic examination of the eye and behavioural tests of vision, complemented by objective investigations (preferential looking, neurophysiological, imaging), establish the nature of the disorder and the severity of the impairment, and indicate a plan for medical treatment and follow-up (see Chapters 2, 3 and 7).

Use of residual/available vision

The assessment of visual function is modified, within a structured format, to suit the presenting status of each baby. The vision necessary for achievement of each developmental goal is assessed in turn. Visual awareness for standard test items nearest in size to the natural learning material and/or for relevant features within the natural environment (*e.g.* floor colouring, room uprights) is observed. If absent, the standard lure is replaced by progressively more visually prominent ones (larger, more colourful, more contrasted). Once a visible lure has been identified, awareness of it within different areas of the visual field and at different distances is explored. The findings are assimilated into practical advice.

The developmental goal for babies B and C described earlier was the ability to locate sound. Baby C understood that the splash meant that the bottle was present and that he could reach out for it, but he was unable to place the sound in space. A developmental paediatrician would explore visual awareness for dangling balls of different size/colour in each area of his visual field within three quarters of a metre. Suppose in the right temporal and central fields he notices an 8cm coloured ball, but in the left temporal field only a strongly contrasted one of at least 18cm diameter within 30cm of his face: parents could be advised that most rattles and everyday items will allow him to learn through his vision in the right and central fields but that he will require much larger, brighter ones closer to him on the left. Baby B had not yet realized the potential of his hands for reaching; his visual assessment would note his awareness of neutral and brightly coloured 5cm balls at 25 to 30cm in his central fields. If aware of the latter but not the former, a pair of brightly coloured gloves might be advised.

Promotion of visual development

As already mentioned, visual development is frequently suboptimal during the biologically critical period for development of neuronal templates within the visual nervous system. One factor may be that visual images received by the cortex of an SVI neonate are too degraded to excite the central driving force of visual development—'looking' to extract meaning. The provision of meaning to what is seen is the first priority of a developmentally based programme to promote visual development. Such a programme has been scientifically evaluated in 58 SVI infants aged 0 to 13 months at outset (Sonksen *et al.* 1991). Over a 12 month period, babies receiving the programme made substantially more progress than controls, including the majority of those with no apparent vision or awareness of light only, and those with additional disabilities; the only visual diagnoses which precluded progress were Norrie's disease and Leber's amaurosis. Response to the programme was equally good when introduced in the second six months of life as in the first; the advantage of early introduction lies in the earlier availability of higher quality vision for general development. Subsequent follow-up suggests that the programme should continue to be updated until progress stops or the ceiling of the programme is reached; also that introduction during the second and third year of life is often rewarded by visual progress.

The assessment is functional and aims to identify visual targets and define distance, arc and speed of movement parameters which can be assimilated into a programme to develop acuity and train neuromotor ocular functions, from near following to distance tracking. 'Looking' is encouraged by reinforcement of early visual experiences through touch and sound; the visual characteristics of developmentally appropriate targets are enhanced as necessary, and concepts and motor skills inherent in early visual behaviours are facilitated. The sequence of developing visual behaviours seen in sighted babies is followed. Details of the programme and methods of visual assessment have been published previously (Sonksen *et al.* 1991).

The preschool era
Once a baby has acquired the basic skills and understanding of a sighted 12- to 15-month-old, progress within individual avenues of development becomes less dependent upon achievement in others. The scheme of assessment needs to embrace the gradual delineation into channels, by seeking to identify which avenues are currently most constrained, and subjecting them to a greater depth of assessment with a view to intervention. The patterns of difficulty within some areas and vulnerability to clinical problems within others often vary with the degree of visual impairment.

Non-verbal concepts
The author has noticed marked differences in the patterns of emergence of concepts of size, shape and colour in babies with different degrees of visual impairment. Obviously, colour cannot become a meaningful concept for children who are totally blind, because unlike shape and size it cannot be learnt through tactile experience. In children with sufficient acuity to distinguish gross features of form, the sequence is similar to that in sighted children—size and shape in tandem followed by colour. In contrast, children with intermediate acuity (awareness only of presence of large near objects) often develop concepts of colour first; many can name them before 3 years of age. The patterns underline the major role normally played by vision in the acquisition of non-verbal concepts.

Development of the tactile sense
Although tactile sensitivity and discrimination (stereognosis) and exploratory scanning strategies hardly feature in developmental debate or assessment and teaching schemes for very young children, they merit serious consideration in those with SVI. In the experience of the DVC team all these skills are poorer during the preschool years in SVI children than in sighted peers; their development, like those of the other senses, is normally tutored by vision and constrained by severe impairment. Children with sufficient vision to discern the presence and gross characteristics of near objects develop visual scanning strategies and, like sighted

people, translate strategic understanding into tactile mode as necessary. In contrast, blind and near-blind children experience great difficulty in acquiring scanning strategies. In the DVC these skills are assessed using structured observation for graded tactile tasks, and interventions are prescribed according to the findings (Sonksen and Stiff 1991). Presumably, as for the other senses, there is a critical period for laying down neuronal templates and networks, so special attention should also be given to the promotion of tactile development in preschool children at risk of becoming blind, *e.g.* those with incomplete retinopathy of prematurity or buphthalmos.

Language development
Reynell (1979) pointed to an unusual pattern of language development in some young children: word combinations in expressive speech perhaps months before comprehension of simple requests. In a retrospective study of 40 otherwise normal 12- to 24-month-old SVI children attending the DVC, McConachie (1990) confirmed this pattern in a third of those with minimal or no perception of light, but did not encounter it amongst those with visually directed reach for large near objects. The latter group were much more likely to exhibit equal levels of comprehension and expression or a two- to three-month expressive delay in comparison with age-matched sighted children. A third of the former (blind) group showed equal levels and a third two to three months expressive delay; the outcome for the latter group at age 2½ to 3 years was mixed—expressive catch-up, general delay and severe expressive disorder. Awareness by the clinician that the 'advanced' expressive pattern does not necessarily truly reflect an SVI child's cognitive functioning is important when considering readiness for nursery (preschool) group placement and when counselling parents about potential. Further studies are needed before outcome for the different groups can be predicted. The influence of differences in patterns of early parent–baby interaction has been investigated by McConachie and Moore (1993). Their study of 16 young SVI children suggested that even a small amount of vision makes a major difference to the parents' ability to understand their child's focus of interest. Rather paradoxically, parents of blind children were less likely to amplify the meaning of their input to the child with an accompanying action, or to describe objects and events in detail. Thus the blind children had less help than the group with some useful vision in making links between early language and the concrete world.

Deceleration and regression of development/behavioural disintegration
The onset of developmental delay, stasis or regression and/or behavioural dis-integration during the second and third years of life in blind or near-blind children has been reported in some conditions causing profound visual impairment—*e.g.* Norrie's disease (Warburg 1966) and Leber's amaurosis (Dekalan 1972, Nickel and Hoyt 1982). Rogers and Newhart-Larson (1989), from a study of 10 boys aged 3 to 7 years (five with Leber's amaurosis, five blind from other causes), suggest

that the onset of autism may be a specific association of Leber's amaurosis, representing a primary disturbance within the CNS rather than a secondary feature of blindness. Of the totally blind children attending the DVC, 31 per cent have shown this phenomenon following a documental period of normal development (personal data, unpublished). In some, cognitive stasis/regression and in others disordered social communication was most prominent; occasionally the latter occurred despite continuing cognitive development. Only one child with minimal vision, and none with vision better than this, have been affected. The range of visual diagnoses was wide and included Leber's amaurosis, Norrie's disease, retinopathy of prematurity, anophthalmia, optic disc hypoplasia and total blindness of unknown cause.

Our experience suggests that this phenomenon is not disorder-specific but a risk in many conditions causing congenital blindness. More than half the DVC children so afflicted had experienced emotionally stressful medical or family events during the second year. The second year encompasses several of the most challenging phases in the development of attention control and independence for a toddler and these will be significantly greater for a blind one. Evidence is accumulating that primary dysgenesis of the CNS is sometimes an association of several of the conditions which give rise to congenital blindness (Goodyear *et al.* 1989, Roberts-Harry *et al.* 1990, Black and Sonksen 1992). Further research is needed to clarify the issues, but an interplay of the above factors is probably responsible for the clinical picture presented by an individual child. Professionals involved in the care of SVI children need to be aware that this is a vulnerable period for a totally blind child, because awareness is the stepping stone to successful prevention and management.

Visual assessment
Regular ophthalmological supervision of the primary eye condition, plus correction of any refractive or amblyopic element to the visual impairment, is essential for all SVI preschool children.

PROMOTION OF VISUAL DEVELOPMENT
Once basic ocular motor mechanisms and visual awareness of objects in the near environment are established, the emphasis of the assessment of visual function for the programme of visual development and the activities prescribed can shift to distance skills and discrimination of details; an example of the latter might be a play activity requiring discrimination of three everyday items of similar overall size, shape and colour but differing in detail, *e.g.* red ball, red apple, red shoe (Sonksen and Stiff 1991, Sonksen *et al.* 1991).

USE OF RESIDUAL/AVAILABLE VISION
Everyday items, scenes and realistic life-size pictures are the learning materials of 15- to 60-month-olds; print and stylized black and white pictures become

increasingly relevant from the age of 54 months but are not the primary learning medium until the second or third year of infant school (6 to 7 years). It is very easy to overestimate a child's vision for everyday objects and pictures because *familiar ones* can be recognized from gross visual clues, such as colour and outline, at much greater distance than that required to identify or learn about them initially. A formal assessment of vision for age-appropriate learning materials therefore can be of considerable value to parents, teachers and therapists working with an SVI child.

A technique to establish three qualitative levels of vision for objects, pictures, colours, print, etc. has been developed by the present author. The vocabulary of younger children requires preliminary exploration using objects dissimilar in colour to those used in the tests.

● *Stage 1*. Pictures from the Sonksen Picture Guide to Visual Function (Sonksen and Macrae 1987) and objects are used. Each test item is presented at 3m, 2m, 1m, 0.5m and <0.5m until correctly identified. The identification distance reflects a child's capacity to resolve fine detail and defines the maximum distance at which s/he can learn from materials of visual complexity similar to that of the test items. If objects not identified visually are named after tactile exploration the assessor has information about the nature of materials that a child cannot resolve visually at any distance.

● *Stage 2*. Some of the child's own toys or belongings, or the now familiar test objects or pictures are then presented in a similar way. The identification distance now reflects a child's capacity to resolve gross visual characteristics and defines the maximum distance at which s/he can recognize familiar objects and pictures of visual complexity similar to the test items. The distance at which a child can recognize different size masses of colour can be established using 10cm, 5cm, 2.5cm and 1.2cm squares of primary colours and a similar test technique (poor colour sensitivity is more often a problem in children with SVI than specific colour defect).

● *Stage 3*. For children with insufficient vision to achieve stage 2, items of different size, colour and luminance are gradually brought nearer until visual awareness is observed; the distance defines the maximum distance of a child's visual awareness for items with gross visual characteristics similar to those of the test item.

The findings are used to prescribe practical guidelines for parents and teachers to use at home and in the classroom. Assessment of fields and best/worse patches of field is an important additional parameter for some children. Many parents, therapists, teachers and paediatricians observing this assessment comment that it helps them understand how the child sees.

Reading becomes the major medium for learning during the infant school years (5 to 11 years); in parallel, writing becomes an important mode of expression. In older children and adults the classification of degree of visual impairment into educational categories is based on a measure of linear acuity according to the Snellen standard. The measurement taken for young SVI children attending eye and paediatric clinics in the UK is frequently single optotype (SO). Personal experience of SVI children aged 3½ to 7 years suggests that the crowding ratio (linear measure : SO measure) is frequently between two and four, *e.g.* linear 6/24, SO 6/9. SO measures may bolster the hopes of parents and testers, but often ill serve an SVI child by overestimating acuity and underestimating problems experienced with reading, so that s/he may be placed in the wrong educational category and be denied the special educational support s/he requires. The same rationale applies to near measures of acuity. A suitable linear test for children is the Sonksen–Silver Acuity System (Sonksen and Silver 1988).

The size of linear display seen at a glance is the measure relevant to daily functioning, not the size achieved after lengthy inspection aided by intelligent guesswork. A description of the former that includes size and distance is a most useful guideline arising from the functional assessment of vision. Similarly, the measure of near acuity of practical value is the size of linear display seen 'easily' at a distance >25cm, a distance which facilitates the breadth of new scanning and allows optimal use of available lighting.

There is a need to take the functional assessment further than 'at a glance' acuity for Snellen displays because the contrast and integral proportions of a child's pencil script will be different and more difficult to see than the former. The examiner writes in pencil in a school exercise book using similar size script to the child's. If the child has difficulty in seeing the examiner's writing, the assessment is continued by increasing the contrast and width of component strokes of letters, *e.g.* by using black felt-tip pens on better quality paper. A firm recommendation based on the finding will ensure that a child is able to monitor her/his own work effectively.

Unlike adults and older children who have lost vision, young children with congenital visual impairment may not appreciate or express their difficulties. These need to be actively sought by the assessment team and addressed individually. Experience and skill on the part of the tester are needed to modify and extend standard test techniques to address a breadth of visual functions, as is a facility to present the findings in the form of practical guidelines meaningful to other disciplines.

Low-vision aids
Traditionally, low-vision aids have been considered for individuals who have lost sight and who can express their needs: preschool children have been thought to be 'too young'. The vision team at The Wolfson Centre have researched their use in preschool children (Ritchie *et al.* 1989). Subsequently, a low-vision aid clinic for young children in which a developmental paediatrician and an ophthalmic optician work jointly with the child and parents has been established (Gould and Sonksen 1991). Developmental levels in language, performance and attention control of sighted 2- to 3-year-olds are sufficient for success with simple stand magnifiers and those of 3- to 4-year-olds for distance telescopes. Sufficient vision to see a 1.5cm sweet or identify a size 12m Snellen optotype at 10cm and a 2cm white ball or a size 60m Snellen optotype at 2m is required before benefit can be expected with a near

magnifier and distance telescope respectively. Children with the lowest levels of vision need to be slightly more developmentally mature to benefit than those with higher levels. Interestingly, 'unaided' visual acuity improved in many children during a six week trial period with the aids, pointing once again to the importance of 'looking for meaning' to the development of visual acuity.

Conclusion

To be born with SVI is a crisis which requires experienced developmental and visual management throughout the early years. The vulnerability of parents and baby varies over time, with degree of visual impairment and within disorders. Visual management requires cooperation between ophthalmic and developmental teams; developmental aspects of visual management include promotion of visual development, use of residual/available vision and low-vision aids.

SVI babies and young children with additional disabilities need a similar approach to assessment and design of developmental and visual intervention. Assessment techniques require even more skilful modification and critical interpretation. Intervention design must encompass the constraints imposed by the additional disabilities as well as the visual ones. An experienced multidisciplinary team which includes all the therapies is essential.

REFERENCES

Black, M.M., Sonksen, P.M. (1992) 'The congenital retinal dystrophies: a study of early cognitive and visual development.' *Archives of Disease in Childhood*, **67**, 262–265.
Dekalan, A.S. (1972) 'Mental retardation and neurologic involvement in patients with congenital retinal blindness.' *Developmental Medicine and Child Neurology*, **14**, 436–444.
Goodyear, H.M., Sonksen, P.M., McConachie, H. (1989) 'Norrie's disease: a prospective study of development.' *Archives of Disease in Childhood*, **64**, 1587–1592.
Gould, E., Sonksen, P.M. (1991) 'A low vision aid clinic for pre-school children.' *British Journal of Visual Impairment*, **9**, 44–45.
McConachie, H. (1990) 'Early language development and severe visual impairment.' *Child: Care Health and Development*, **16**, 55–61.
—— Moore, V. (1993) 'Early expressive language of severely visually impaired children.' *Developmental Medicine and Child Neurology. (In press.)*
McKendrick, O. (1991) *Assessment of Multi-handicapped Visually Impaired Children.* London: RNIB.
Nickel, B., Hoyt, C.S. (1982) 'Leber's congenital amaurosis. Is mental retardation a frequent associated defect?' *Archives of Ophthalmology*, **100**, 1089–1092.
Reynell, J. (1979) *Reynell–Zinkin Developmental Scales for Visually Handicapped Children. Part I, Mental Development.* Windsor, Berkshire: NFER.
Ritchie, J.P., Sonksen, P.M., Gould, E. (1989) 'Low vision aids for preschool children.' *Developmental Medicine and Child Neurology*, **31**, 509–519.
Roberts-Harry, J., Green, S.H., Willshaw, H.E. (1990) 'Optic nerve hypoplasia: associations and management.' *Archives of Disease in Childhood*, **65**, 103–106.
Rogers, S.J., Newhart-Larson, S. (1989) 'Characteristics of infantile autism in five children with Leber's congenital amaurosis.' *Developmental Medicine and Child Neurology*, **31**, 598–608.
Sonksen, P.M. (1983a) 'The assessment of "Vision for Development" in severely visually handicapped babies.' *Acta Ophthalmologica*, **157**, (Suppl.), 82–91.
—— (1983b) 'Vision and early development.' *In:* Wybar, K., Taylor, D. (Eds) *Paediatric Ophthalmology: Current Aspects.* New York: Marcel Dekker, pp. 85–94.

—— (1989) 'Constraints upon parenting: experience of a paediatrician.' *Child: Care, Health and Development*, **15**, 29–36.

—— Macrae, A.J. (1987) 'Vision for coloured pictures at different acuities: the Sonksen Picture Guide to Visual Function.' *Developmental Medicine and Child Neurology*, **29**, 337–347.

—— Silver, J. (1988) *The Sonksen–Silver Acuity System: Instruction Manual.* Windsor, Berkshire: Keeler.

—— Stiff, B. (1991) *Show Me What My Friends Can See: A Developmental Guide for Parents of Babies with Severely Impaired Sight and their Professional Advisers.* London: Institute of Child Health.

—— Levitt, S.L., Kitzinger, M. (1984) 'Identification of constraints acting on motor development in young visually disabled children and principles of remediation.' *Child: Care, Health and Development*, **10**, 273–286.

—— Petrie, A., Drew, K.J. (1991) 'Promotion of visual development in severely visually impaired babies: evaluation of a developmentally based programme.' *Developmental Medicine and Child Neurology*, **33**, 320–335.

Warburg, M. (1966) 'Norrie's disease; a congenital progessive occulo-accoustico-cerebral degeneration.' *Acta Ophthalmologica*, **89** (Suppl.), 1–147.

7
OPHTHALMIC MANAGEMENT

Alistair R. Fielder

Many clinicians feel ill at ease with the management of the infant or child with visual impairment (VI). Perhaps because the magnitude, permanence and untreatability of the visual deficit inevitably dominate the picture, it can be difficult for the clinician to appreciate that s/he has an important positive role. This is incorrect, as there is much to do.

In the absence of a substantial body of literature, this chapter will be a largely personal account. Although written from the ophthalmic and medical viewpoint, hopefully it will be relevant to all clinical and non-clinical disciplines. Ophthalmic details have been kept to a minimum.

Organization of health, education and other professional services varies both within and between countries, and this chapter will deal mainly with concepts rather than details of management.

Attitudes

Anyone exposed to patient support groups, or voluntary organizations dealing with people with VI, cannot fail to be aware of the mixed attitudes toward the medical profession. It is so fundamental that the carer be sensitive to patient and parental attitudes that some space will be devoted to this issue.

Dr William Silverman, active in neonatal research during the epidemic of blindness due to retinopathy of prematurity in the late 1940s, can introduce this topic. Later he obtained the views of some of the survivors of this period and their parents (Silverman 1980), paraphrased recently in the *Lancet* (1991):

Most of the parents harboured bitterness towards their doctors, not for failure to anticipate the disastrous effects of oxygen therapy but for their apparent indifference to their plight. This is an appalling indictment of medical behaviour that the profession cannot afford to ignore.

Unfortunately these comments are still pertinent to today's practice. A recent survey on the needs of the visually disabled child (Walker *et al.* 1992), reported that for around 80 per cent of parents their major complaint was lack of information, mainly on medical topics. Clearly there has been no substantial improvement in attitudes and communication over the past four decades.

What does this mean in the context of childhood VI? Parents usually recognize that not all blindness can be prevented, that certain conditions are not amenable to treatment, and that treatment outcome is not always successful. They also appreciate the need for medical input into the management of VI at a variety of levels. However, they resent the defensive attitudes and apparent lack of interest in their plight shown by the medical profession.

Both parents and professionals can experience difficulty in openly discussing the complex issues surrounding VI. The parent's reactions can range from helplessness to anger and frustration—emotions readily understood, but less easily coped with, by the professional, partly because of a poor understanding of VI.

The basis of clinical defensiveness is complicated. First, the failure to eliminate, or even reduce, the VI induces feelings of inadequacy. Second, not appreciating that this 'failure' is often understood by the family could result in an inability to communicate openly with them. Third, techniques have not permitted the clinician to quantify visual functions in early childhood. Indeed, our understanding of the natural history of visual pathway disorders is so poor that clinicians are often not prepared to venture an opinion for fear of being incorrect. This is understandable, as the consequence of misplaced optimism is far more damaging than that of undue pessimism. Fourth, many of the clinical parameters of vision bear little relation to functional ability.

One suggestion to facilitate clinical understanding of the reality of VI is to answer the question, for each clinical situation, '*What does this visual disorder mean to the child and her/his family: now and for the future?*' Clearly it would be arrogant and patronizing for the clinician to presume to know the answer to this question. However, the attempt is worthwhile, as it requires a knowledge of the effects of the disorder on everyday functions, the implications for family life, the future prognosis and the genetic implications, if any.

Trite examples of 'what does it mean to me?' are given in Figure 7.1. Figure 7.1*a* was presented to three sighted students who were asked the question, 'How would a blind person see this picture?' One said the blind person would see nothing, the second drew Figure 7.1*b* and the third Figure 7.1*c*. The comment by the first child that blind children see nothing at all is a common misconception. The second only considered the objects of interest, which became defocused, and ignored the background. The third decided that not only the objects of interest, but the entire visual field would be affected. This example should not be taken too seriously, but it does indicate that opinions differ on what blind people can see, and that the severity of VI may differ.

Frankly, our ignorance of VI is such that for only a very few conditions can these questions be fully answered. Nevertheless, the exercise is worth doing in an attempt to gain a fresh, empathetic approach, to appreciate what information is required, and to avoid resorting to a well-rehearsed 'patter'.

Hopefully, the professional will enable the parents to achieve that delicate balance between accepting a most difficult situation, and adopting a positive approach to maximize their child's potential—a balance exemplified in this quotation from the mother of a child who, three months after a normal neonatal period, became very severely neurologically damaged and totally blind: 'I'll do anything I can to help, but she's great as she is.'

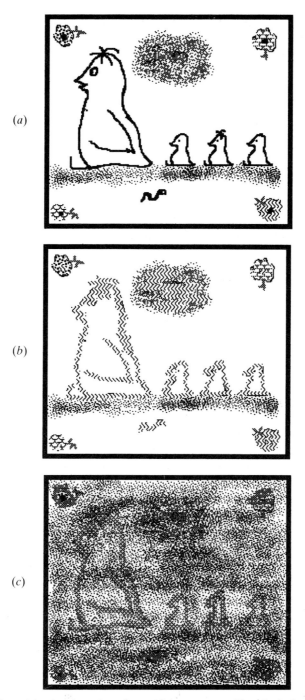

Fig. 7.1. (*a*) Three sighted students were shown this computer graphic and asked to alter it to show what a blind person would see. One drew (*b*), another (*c*), while the third said the blind person would see nothing.

Ophthalmic assessment

Over the past two decades, techniques for evaluating visual pathway function in childhood have advanced considerably. Although all tests have limitations, they have provided valuable insight, unobtainable by traditional methods, into the various patterns of visual functions in visual pathway disorders (see Chapter 3). Reappraisal is essential, as the depth of visual impairment may not be stable, and part of the challenge of management is to monitor and understand any changes of function.

Functional vision

The scene for this topic is best set by the following statement made by a severely visually impaired man: 'Ophthalmologists tell me what I can see, but it doesn't bear much relation to what I can do.' Similar comments are frequently heard from clients and non-medical professionals, and they cast doubt on the relevance to everyday function of traditional parameters of vision such as distance and near visual acuity, colour vision and the visual field. For instance, distance acuity does not correlate well with educational performance. Near acuity is a somewhat better indicator, and sustained reading correlates better with educational performance. The standard method of testing near vision, with a few words from a text which might be held in an awkward position, might be difficult to maintain over a period of time. In contrast, the sustained reading test involves the reading of all of a preselected passage of a few hundred words (Dickinson and Rabbitt 1991, Leat and Woodhouse 1992) and therefore simulates closer the real life situation. The relevance of recording contrast sensitivity is also uncertain in the context of VI. Using black and white stripes as an example, contrast sensitivity is the measure of blackness and whiteness, whereas in VI the distinction may be less well defined, resulting in greyness or 'fogging'. This is important, for instance, when considering the lighting environment of the visually impaired schoolchild. However, in practice the quantification of contrast sensitivity appears to be of less value than understanding the basic concept. The relevance to function of visual field defects, such as hemianopias, peripheral constriction, central and paracentral scotomata, are better understood.

The terms functional, useful, or 'real' vision indicate the vision necessary for everyday leisure, educational or workplace activity. Inevitably, the functional vision required varies for different activities. Apart from certain obvious influences on activities such as visual field defects and night blindness, the quotation above indicates that the concepts and parameters of functional vision are poorly understood. Research is obviously called for, but for now the clinician should not consider that standard ophthalmic parameters accurately predict function.

To summarize, although the precise relation of ophthalmic parameters to functional vision is unknown, certain of these should be measured or considered: visual acuity (distance and near), colour vision, the visual field, and possibly contrast sensitivity (see above).

Patterns of presentation

Not all visual impairment in childhood presents dramatically. Recognition of the various patterns of presentation is important for management, to reduce delay in the institution of support, and to ensure only the appropriate involvement of other disciplines. Some of these clinical patterns of presentations will now be discussed.

Dramatic presentation

A dramatic presentation of VI is readily understood and is accompanied by great parental concern. The obvious example is the infant with absent or reduced visual responses due to a retinal disorder (*e.g.* Leber's amaurosis), or optic nerve abnormality (*e.g.* optic nerve hypoplasia). An older child may also present dramatically with sudden loss of vision due to a severe neurological catastrophe, such as a cerebral tumour. Because reduced vision is the dominant feature, infants and children in this category usually present first to the ophthalmologist.

Creeping presentation

The term 'creeping' covers VI which is unnoticed or overlooked due to preoccupation with other aspects of medical care. This does not reflect a disinterest in welfare, but indicates rather the complexity of paediatric–ophthalmic evaluation. It is a trivial title, used more for its sense than for accuracy. However, it is defended, because this type of presentation is quite common, and is important, because failure to recognize the VI may cause long delays in service delivery.

OCULAR DISORDERS UNDERGOING TREATMENT

Surprisingly, active ophthalmic treatment can delay the initiation of VI support (unpublished personal observations). Three obvious examples are infantile glaucoma, the cataracts of Still's disease and retinopathy of prematurity (ROP), all of which can cause VI. In the first this can be due to high refractive error, amblyopia, glaucomatous damage or systemic associations such as Down syndrome. In the second, when cataract surgery is required the outlook for normal vision is very remote, and VI likely. With severe ROP, many ophthalmic examinations will have been undertaken in the neonatal period, and probably treatment performed before VI is recognized. Under these circumstances it is all too easy to concentrate on ROP management and to fail to appreciate that meanwhile the infant has become visually impaired and needs support.

NEUROLOGICAL DISORDERS

Rare in routine ophthalmic practice, a neurodegenerative disorder such as Batten's disease may cause a slow reduction of vision before neurological signs and symptoms become apparent. The child with sudden vision loss, as for instance following an acute rise in intracranial pressure, may not complain of loss of vision. In both examples, symptoms and signs can be misinterpreted and sometimes incorrectly diagnosed as functional blindness (Taylor 1990). Loss of vision should be considered in the child with recently altered or atypical behaviour. Poor vision in the child with severe learning difficulties may also pass unnoticed.

'Unsuspected' visual impairment

Poor vision may well have been observed but considered simply to be part of a generalized problem (*e.g.* neurodevelopmental delay, learning difficulties), and not necessarily a reason for evaluating visual function. However, identifying the visual deficit is still important, over and above the standard developmental assessment, to ensure the appropriate support and stimulation to meet individual needs. It should also be stated that in some children with neurodevelopmental delay, severe visual defects are indeed unsuspected. In contrast to dramatic forms of presentation, children in whom VI is 'unsuspected' are usually seen first by the paediatrician rather than the ophthalmologist.

Temporary visual impairment

A number of infants presenting with a severe visual deficit fully recover (Type 1 delayed visual maturation—see below). Clearly under these circumstances the involvement of VI services is not required and might be an unnecessary worry for the parents. The features which differentiate delayed visual maturation from permanent causes of VI have been discussed by Tresidder *et al.* (1990) and Fielder and Mayer (1991) and will not be considered here.

Potential visual impairment

This group includes the infant or child suffering a serious ophthalmic condition with the potential for causing VI. Rather than leaving the parents uninformed, visual development should be repeatedly quantified. Prediction carries certain dangers (outlined below); nevertheless, the acuity value given at each visit describes the development to date and may help parents understand progress. Furthermore, if acuity is normal, or near normal, the clinician can allay the parents' worst fears very early. Conversely, when the visual deficit is severe, rehabilitation can be commenced immediately.

Patterns of visual development

Providing advice on vision is fraught with difficulty, and this section is included to emphasize that vision, even in the visually impaired child, may not be stable, and because some comprehension of the various patterns of development is essential for adequate counselling. As yet our understanding of these patterns is still rudimentary.

Two well known ophthalmic adages set the scene: 'Never tell a parent her/his infant is blind, you may be wrong'; 'Beware of telling the parent of an infant thought to be blind that improvement may occur, for if incorrect, this will cause far more distress than if you had not attempted to make a forecast.'

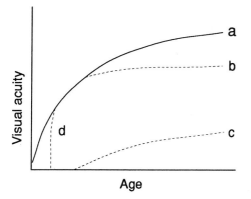

Fig. 7.2. Normal visual development (line a). Early delayed visual development with rapid (line d) and slow incomplete improvement (line c). The line (a) pattern is seen in delayed visual maturation type 1, and (c) in some children with Leber's amaurosis and other conditions. Asymptotic or plateau patterns (line b) are found in congenital/infantile nystagmus. These figures all indicate the difficulty of predicting future visual development.

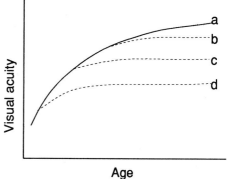

Fig. 7.3. Asymptotic visual development. The level at which plateauing occurs depends on the severity of the visual pathway abnormality.

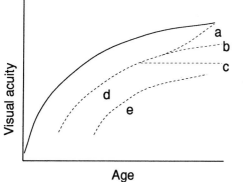

Fig. 7.4. Parallel visual development, seen in aphakia and severe retinopathy of prematurity. (Also shown is late catch-up, not relevant to visual impairment.)

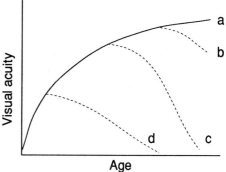

Fig. 7.5. Regression. This occurs in a range of progressive ophthalmic and neurological conditions.

These two contradictory statements will preclude information being passed on to the parent for months, if not years. Although they generate intense parental dissatisfaction, both are based on sound clinical observations but deficient understanding of the natural history of visual pathway disorders. It is implicit in these statements that the clinician cannot confidently predict the pattern for an individual. This is unsurprising, as clinically applicable techniques for measuring

TABLE 7.1

Delayed visual maturation (DVM): subtypes

Type 1: DVM as an isolated anomaly.
　　　　Complete and rapid improvement within the first six months of life

Type 2: DVM with obvious and persistent neurodevelopmental problems.
　　　　Limited improvement, often taking many months

Type 3: DVM associated with infantile nystagmus and albinism.
　　　　Rapid, but incomplete, improvement within six months

Type 4: DVM with severe congenital, bilateral structural ocular abnormalities (excluding albinism).
　　　　Very limited improvement, in some children only

---

vision in infants and young children have only become generally available in the past decade. Not denying the value of electrophysiology, the tests referred to here, which have provided so much information on normal and abnormal development, are preferential looking based tests, notably the acuity card procedure which is simple to administer and can be used as frequently as required. Preferential looking based tests have increased our understanding of visual pathway disorders and have revealed certain patterns of visual development (Fielder *et al.* 1992), as shown in Figures 7.2 to 7.5.

Early infancy
Acuity development in early infancy may be normal, delayed or stationary.

DELAYED EARLY DEVELOPMENT
Reduced or absent visual responsiveness which is present from birth but later improves is termed delayed visual maturation (DVM) (Tresidder *et al.* 1990, Fielder and Mayer 1991). Once considered a single entity, it is now recognized as a broad spectrum. At present four subtypes are known (Table 7.1).

In contrast to Type 1 DVM, in Types 2 and 4 improvement is limited by neurological and ocular pathology respectively. Type 4 DVM is particularly perplexing, as limited improvement of vision *may* occur in infants or young children with severe and permanent structural disorders such as Leber's amaurosis, optic nerve hypoplasia or coloboma.

STATIONARY IMPAIRMENT
In many individuals impaired vision remains stable throughout life, as in total disorganization of the interior of the eye by fibrovascular tissue, or persistent hyperplastic primary vitreous and advanced ROP.

Later visual development
Certain patterns of visual acuity development later in infancy and early childhood have also been recognized.

ASYMPTOTIC VISUAL DEVELOPMENT

Visual development may not achieve normal levels, but plateau at an early stage. This asymptotic (plateauing) pattern may follow normal or delayed early development, and the level at which the plateau occurs depends on the severity of the abnormality. For example, the vision of an infant with a large macular lesion due to toxoplasmosis may develop normally for the first three or so months of life, but then stabilize at around 6/60. Exemplifying the asymptotic pattern following delayed early visual development, a child with albinism may have no visual response in early infancy but then show subsequent improvement, only to plateau later (Tresidder *et al.* 1990).

PARALLEL VISUAL DEVELOPMENT

In this pattern, acuity parallels normal development, albeit at a subnormal level. It is seen in aphakia and severe ROP.

'CATCH-UP' VISUAL DEVELOPMENT

In the various types of DVM after visual unresponsiveness, there is a catch-up phase, although this is not complete in all types.

REGRESSION

Deterioration can follow any of the above developmental patterns due to a wide range of ophthalmic and neurological conditions, including inflammatory eye disease, neurodegenerative disorders, cerebral tumours and intracranial compressive lesions.

Does knowledge of the patterns of development help management?

Perhaps now defensive clinical attitudes are more understandable! Only recently has it become possible to measure vision in infants and young children. Visual development can be monitored and parents updated frequently. However, predicting future development is fraught with difficulty as the various patterns described above are only just being defined.

The following are three frequently encountered clinical situations.

● *Eye totally disorganized by fibrovascular tissue, or anophthalmia.* This is one situation when improvement cannot occur. Although vitrectomy can often successfully remove the fibrovascular tissue (in advanced ROP, for example), the outcome for vision is dismal (Quinn *et al.* 1991).

● *Severe structural ocular abnormality such as retinal dystrophy (Leber's amaurosis), coloboma, optic nerve abnormality, etc.* Surprisingly, improvement does occasionally occur in the presence of severe ocular abnormalities (Type 4 DVM—Fielder and Mayer 1991, Fielder *et al.* 1991), but if it does it is very limited, *i.e.* the child may gain navigational vision but remain legally blind. Unfortunately there are no features which permit the clinician to distinguish the child who will or will not improve. It is therefore not recommended that improvement is openly predicted, for if incorrect, it would cause unnecessary and severe parental disappointment.

• *Blind infant with normal eye findings and a normal electroretinogram.* This large group, in which a retinal cause of blindness has been excluded, contains the many forms of DVM and cortical blindness. If visual loss is the sole abnormality and there is no neurodevelopmental impairment, the prognosis for vision is good (see above). In the presence of a neurodevelopmental or ocular problem, the prognosis is not so good and the clinician should be very cautious.

Deterioration can only be anticipated with knowledge of the pathological process.

These examples illustrate the need to understand both the nature of the visual pathway disorder and its natural history. It is now apparent that vision may improve in *some* conditions previously considered stationary; indeed, only in totally disorganized eyes can it categorically be stated that vision will never improve. The importance of being cautious about predicting future development is again emphasized.

Periods of childhood visual impairment

The management of childhood VI involves many medical and non-medical disciplines. A major problem facing professionals is avoiding either insufficient care or a surfeit of inappropriate involvement. Needs alter during childhood, and it is helpful to subdivide childhood into periods, as this gives the opportunity for all parties to consider what has been done and what remains to be done. These are flexible, not rigid, guidelines. These periods have different implications for the child, parent, teacher, physician, social worker, etc.

Period 1: Presentation and diagnosis

Whatever the mode of presentation, this is medically one of the most challenging periods of ophthalmic management and can be subdivided into various sections.

AROUND THE TIME OF PRESENTATION

• *Making a diagnosis and determining the extent of the visual deficit.* This is both clinically demanding and critical, with pressure to make a diagnosis and determine the extent of the VI as speedily as possible. Despite the new techniques mentioned above, determining the extent of the visual deficit can still be difficult or even impossible. If the necessary equipment and facilities are to hand (*e.g.* acuity cards and electrophysiology), this can often be undertaken in one or two visits, although further investigation, with referral to other medical and/or ophthalmic specialists, may be necessary.

• *What should be said?* Even without a diagnosis, parents and carers will want as much information as possible, and as soon as possible. This is how it should be, and communications should always be open. Patients and parents of patients usually accept that the full details of the case cannot always be determined immediately.

Parents should be given the opportunity to air concerns. Even without a diagnosis, the visual status can be given, and many fears may be laid to rest by stating that certain serious conditions have been eliminated, *e.g.* a tumour in the eye.

One should attempt to quantify (this word is used advisedly) visual functions: there is far more to functional vision than acuity alone. Parents should be given as much information as possible, and it can be helpful to explain the concept of functional vision. The complex patterns of visual development described need to be borne in mind when predicting future development.

• *Review*. One of the most hurtful methods of dealing with a family is to make a diagnosis, give what information is considered necessary, possibly register the infant or child as blind, and then arrange for a review six months ahead, or worse not at all, because 'nothing can be done'. Sadly this still occurs, and unsurprisingly the family dealt with in such a way feel resentful and abandoned.

After the first visit, the parents will have many questions and should be seen again within a very short time (not exceeding two weeks). Local circumstances dictate frequency, and if the first visit has been at a major centre far from home, personal review may not be possible, in which case arrangements closer to home should be made.

The purpose of this first review visit is to clarify issues raised previously and also to undertake further investigations as necessary.

• *Other medical opinions*. As the majority of children with VI have problems additional to their visual defect (see Chapter 1), every visually impaired infant and child should be under paediatric care. VI also has implications for general development, the effects of which may be minimized by appropriate stimulation. The paediatrican is often the best placed member of the medical profession to supervise overall care (see Chapter 8), as s/he has the best working knowledge of the range of paediatric medical and non-medical services. The precise designation of that paediatrician depends on local circumstances, but s/he should be aware of both the associations and the developmental implications of VI and the limitations of her/his expertise (O'Sullivan *et al.* 1992).

Other medical opinions may be required to complete investigations. The need for a further ophthalmic opinion may be considered for a number of reasons. The diagnosis may be uncertain. It may also be requested by parents, particularly in a relatively small centre. Whatever the feelings of the clinician at this juncture, s/he should be sensitive to the parents, who have just had many hopes for the future of their child dashed. Finally, recognizing the consequences of the diagnosis, a further 'back-up' opinion might be suggested by the clinician. Instead of waiting for a request by parents, a clinician-initiated proposal for another opinion can defuse any tension which might have been generated. This is simply an indication of clinical openness and sets the scene well for future care.

• *Who else should be involved?* The management of the VI child requires the involvement of a number of professionals: paediatrician, family doctor, orthoptist, optometrist, peripatetic and other teachers for the sighted and visually impaired, generic and specialist social worker, educational psychologist, rehabilitation and mobility officers, etc. This long list is incomplete, and the relative importance of each profession will depend on local circumstances and traditions. More important, the value of each of these individuals will vary during the different periods of life. As the ophthalmologist is often the identifier of the VI it is essential that s/he is acquainted with local arrangements, as inappropriate initial contact can set off a chain of events resulting in excessive, or inadequate, involvement. To avoid this trap, local protocols need to be drawn up. Each professional should know how to make contact with the key person who understands the range of local services, and in turn is able to liaise with the VI team (see below). The need for a multidisciplinary approach is highlighted by a recent report showing that advice given by paediatricians on health issues was considered useful, whereas much of that related to the disability and to personal and family needs was not (O'Sullivan *et al.* 1992).

• *Vision impairment team*. With the need to coordinate services, certain areas have created VI teams. This was recommended in the UK over two decades ago by the Vernon Committee (1972), who raised the idea of the key worker (named person) within the team who would act as the point of contact for the family and liaise with other services. Unfortunately, in many areas services for the visually impaired are still woefully disjointed and there is no forum for multidisciplinary discussion. There is little doubt that multidisciplinary VI teams do perform an important function. They fall into two broad categories according to local needs: assessment and administrative. In assessment teams, members clinically evaluate children and come together for discussion. Administrative teams discuss the service provision for all visually impaired children in an area, develop local protocols, and while individual children are not seen, they can be discussed: members ensure that 'everything that can be done is done'. Every visually impaired infant or child should be referred as soon as possible to the local VI team, if one exists.

• *Communication*. Failures of communication by clinicians, and ophthalmologists in particular, are a major cause for discontent expressed by parents and non-ophthalmic professionals.

(a) Parents and the family.

The need for verbal communication at all stages is vital: defensiveness can easily be sensed and engenders distrust. As mentioned, the clinician should acknowledge what is unknown to medical science and also the limitations of her/his personal expertise.

Providing written information should be considered. This comes in two forms: specific to the ophthalmic condition, and general on the management of the visually impaired child. Pamphlets are useful for certain conditions, such as strabismus or congenital cataract. However, many causes of VI are rare, and prepared pamphlets cannot cover every eventuality. One alternative is for the clinician to write to the parents after a consultation. Initially the letter may be relatively limited, taking care not to raise new topics at this juncture. However, it gives parents something to read away from the clinic, and is personal to their child. If a preliminary letter is sent after the first visit, ideally it should be followed up by a more detailed missive later on, when more information is to hand. Prepared pamphlets are perhaps more relevant at this time. Excellent booklets giving general information on the management of the visually impaired child are available (*e.g.* Sonksen and Stiff 1991).

(b) Other professionals.

Confidentiality should be observed, but so long as prior permission is sought from the parents, information can be transferred between relevant professionals. Parents rarely object to the sharing of information which will help their child. Of course the catch here is 'information which will help', which means functional vision. Non-medical professionals are less interested in precise diagnoses than functional aspects and prognosis. Unfortunately, few communications cover information on function.

The case conference is a well established forum for communication between professionals and parents. However, because of the time involved and the geographical separation of specialists, attendance by all disciplines its not always possible, particularly for ophthalmologists. If attendance is not possible, written information can be submitted.

● *Registration as visually impaired (partially sighted/blind)*. In certain countries this is mandatory. Local arrangements influence the process of registration, although registration does not always influence the availability of services to visually impaired children. In the UK, registration does carry some benefits to the child and family and should be considered as a positive step to facilitate support. If explained in this way, parents' reluctance for their child to be so 'labelled' usually subsides. Registration is a means of collecting data on VI.

Although registration should be regarded as a positive action, timing is important. Unless specifically requested by parents, it would be most insensitive to propose registration until a degree of rapport has been established with the family, as it is still regarded by many, albeit incorrectly, as a final irreversible and negative act.

EARLY ON

The clinician needs to review the situation soon after diagnosis. Identifying a visually disabling condition and making the diagnosis is only a small part of the ophthalmic role. At presentation, or soon after, the family will want information on prognosis and the possibilities for treatment. The range of available ophthalmic support is discussed later. However well the clinician considers s/he has communicated with the family, it is useful, and often salutary, to ask the parents for their account of the information given to date. This provides an opportunity to emphasize certain points and fill in gaps, an exercise worth undertaking from time to time during childhood to prevent topics being overlooked.

Visual functions which may not be stable should be quantified and monitored, so that accurate information can be relayed to the family and carers, and the effects of any interventions measured. Furthermore, only by the careful monitoring of vision can knowledge of visual pathway disorders advance and management improve.

As the child will now have been evaluated on a number of occasions, the clinician should have a greater understanding of the nature and prognosis of the condition. If registration has not been considered, and the child is eligible, now is a time to broach the subject.

Many disorders have a genetic basis (see Chapter 1), and because of the rapid advances in this field, referral to a geneticist should be offered. It is important that the ophthalmologist does not provide unsolicited *directive* advice on genetic issues.

Period 2: Preschool

As most childhood VI commences by early infancy, the child should already be well known to all involved and most of the important topics will have been covered. From time to time one should review all the areas discussed above, to see if any relevant items have been omitted.

The most effective method of ensuring that 'everything that can be done is done' is through the VI team. Vested interests abound in the management of VI, which is unsurprising with the large range of disciplines involved and the blurred and changing professional boundaries. The potential for interdisciplinary conflict is likely to remain, but can be minimized by meeting face to face as team members.

Much interest at this time is focused on preparation for formal schooling. Again, the key issue is information transfer on functional vision. It must be remembered that a number of factors other than vision influence the placement of a child into a particular school. Professional boundaries should be respected: it is not appropriate for the ophthalmologist to state which school a particular child should attend, although s/he may sometimes be asked to comment on a disputed placement.

Period 3: School

It is not infrequent for visually impaired children to be discharged from ophthalmic follow-up at a young age because 'there is nothing to do'. In this writer's view, that is incorrect. Visual functions may change and should be monitored as a basis for counselling. Ophthalmic support, including counselling, may be required. If discharged, the child's family naturally sense a lack of commitment and feel abandoned. For all these reasons periodic review should be undertaken.

Many children benefit greatly from optical or technical aids. Aids which are helpful at school should also be provided at home. Ophthalmic support will be discussed below.

Period 4: After school

This is a time of changing occupation and increasing social independence, and management must rise to these new demands. In addition to the topics covered already there are certain issues particularly pertinent to this period.

Due to the different natural history of visual pathway disorders, progress should be reviewed. Because many young adults have long been discharged from ophthalmic departments, it is not uncommon for them to hold several important misconceptions about their disorder which need to be discussed. Frequent areas of concern include the options for treatment, the possibility of deterioration, and whether there are genetic implications.

SUPPORT AND TREATMENT

All aspects of support should be reviewed. New optical aids may be required. Issues concerned with training, rehabilitation and mobility should all be addressed. Hopefully the VI team will still act as the liaison group, but if not, it is up to the individual professional to make his/her own contacts on behalf of the client. Health issues should not be neglected. Visually impaired individuals experience difficulty in gaining adequate exercise through the usual avenues of sport. Because the early symptoms of certain disorders are visually dependent, identification of a serious medical condition by the individual may be delayed. While this is more relevant to the elderly in the identification of haematuria and melaena, sighted carers should be aware of this potential problem.

GENETICS

If genetic counselling has already been undertaken, one should still consider the need for an update, in view of the rapidity of advances in the field. Part of the process of genetic counselling includes a meticulous clinical examination and checking that the original diagnosis is still correct.

Overview

It is now appropriate to give an overview of the ophthalmic (only) management of the VI infant and child. The division of childhood into four periods is helpful, but should not be regarded too rigidly.

The ophthalmic role: assessment

As many of the functions described below can, and often are, undertaken by a range of professionals, such as paediatricians, ophthalmologists, orthoptists and optometrists, the word ophthalmic does not always have strict professional connotations.

MAKING AND CHECKING THE DIAGNOSIS

One of the pivotal ophthalmic duties is to establish the diagnosis. In the light of advances, a diagnosis made in infancy may need to be modified. This may have important implications for prognosis and genetics.

Visual functions should be quantified and monitored. Parents and carers need to know the severity of the visual deficit and what the future holds for visual development. Quantifying vision also opens up the issue of functional vision and its relevance to everyday leisure and work activities.

Although permanent VI by definition cannot be cured, there may well be a treatable element, vital to minimize the degree of impairment and maximize visual potential. This requires accurate knowledge of the function and patterns of development.

LINK PERSON

It is paramount that every ophthalmologist recognizes the importance of a multidisciplinary approach to the management of VI (Gieser 1992) and the value of the contribution of other professionals. Effective care is probably best achieved through the VI team and the named person who has a key role in involving appropriate agencies. The need for maintained involvement of a developmental paediatrician has been emphasized, as has the need to offer genetic counselling if relevant.

REGISTRATION AS VISUALLY IMPAIRED

The need for registration is governed by local arrangements. In those countries with registration, its value as the triggering event for support should not be overlooked.

BEING APPROACHABLE

Problems with approachability remain a constant and major complaint against the medical profession. This is a question of attitude as much as availability. Because of the frequent difficulty in contacting clinicians, one should consider offering parents a simple, direct method of contact by phone, such as at home, or out of hours in the office.

The ophthalmic role: treatment

The role of treatment has not been considered so far as it applies to all periods of childhood and beyond. The word treatment is used to cover specific advice to maximize visual function, in addition to optical and surgical forms of treatment.

GENERAL

Function at home, in the classroom, and also at work, is of paramount importance and should be catered for. An unusual posture, habit, etc. may be a useful adaptive phenomenon by the child to the visual deficit. This fact should be made known to the carers, who sometimes misinterpret these actions as simple mannerisms, although this view is unlikely with those experienced in working with visually impaired children.

Illumination and contrast should not be ignored, as certain individuals function better in dim light (*e.g.* achromatopsia), while others need good lighting conditions and function poorly when light is dim (*e.g.* retinitis pigmentosa). Increasing the level of contrast may improve reading performance for some. Glare can be a problem in a number of conditions. Distance and near acuity levels dictate the optimal position for blackboard work and explain why a child has to hold reading matter very close to the eyes.

Certain children (*e.g.* those with nystagmus and visual field defects) adopt an abnormal head position in order to maximize vision. The beneficial effect of such postures should be recognized, as they may reduce blur and increase acuity, and therefore they should not be discouraged. The child's position in the classroom may need to be altered to accommodate this adaptive habit.

OPTICAL CORRECTION

The importance of optical correction by spectacles and low vision aids (LVAs) cannot be overemphasized. Periodic re-evaluation should be undertaken to meet changing requirements. Although LVAs are expensive, they are simply tools to be used rather than cherished objects. Damage will inevitably occur in the rough and tumble of childhood. Indeed, a child may modify the LVA to maximize its usefulness, which should not be criticized or penalized. If useful at school and work, LVAs should also be available at home.

Tints in spectacles or contact lenses can be vital to optimize visual functions particularly for the child with albinism or achromatopsia. A variety of tint strengths for spectacles may be required to cope with different lighting conditions.

Other technical aids such as closed circuit TV are discussed elsewhere in this book.

Although requirements at home, school and workplace may differ to a degree, the concept of a 'high tech' school and a 'low tech' home is fundamentally unacceptable, taking into account the amount of time spent in the latter. In addition, the relative isolation of the visually impaired child at home, the length of weekends and vacations, and the lack of available outdoor activities all indicate the need for a stimulating home environment.

SURGERY

Ophthalmic surgery may be considered for functional and cosmetic reasons. Both are important and are further reasons for occasional ophthalmic review.

VISUAL STIMULATION

This is much practised, especially with children with neurological deficits. Quantitative data on the natural history of visual pathway disorders have only recently been reported (Fielder *et al.* 1992), and the value of stimulation has yet to be fully determined, although there is one encouraging recent report (Black and Sonksen 1992). Space does not permit further consideration of this topic.

Conclusion

This chapter is a brief overview of the ophthalmic management of the visually impaired infant and child—perhaps rather anecdotal and personal, but the details are less important than the concepts. The ophthalmologist should adopt a positive approach and recognize that there is much to do to help the visually impaired child. It is apparent that very little is known about visual function in VI and its relevance to everyday life. In addition, the management of childhood VI is fragile and depends to a great extent on parental drive and the initiative of individual professionals. Hopefully in the future this will become more robust with the development of protocols and the widespread adoption of professional multi-disciplinary teams who are closer to understanding *what it means to the child and her/his family: now and for the future*.

REFERENCES

Black, M.M., Sonksen, P.M. (1992) 'Congenital retinal dystrophies: a study of early cognitive and visual development.' *Archives of Disease in Childhood*, **67**, 262–265.

Dickinson, C.M., Rabbitt, P.M.A. (1991) 'Simulated visual impairment: effects on text comprehension and reading speed.' *Clinical Vision Science*, **6**, 301–308.

Fielder, A.R., Mayer, D.L. (1991) 'Delayed visual maturation'. *Seminars in Ophthalmology*, **6**, 182–193.

—— Fulton, A.B., Mayer, D.L. (1991) 'Visual development of infants with severe ocular disorders.' *Ophthalmology*, **98**, 1306–1309.

—— Dobson, V., Moseley, M.J., Mayer, D.L. (1992) 'Preferential looking—clinical lessons.' *Ophthalmic Paediatrics and Genetics*, **13**, 101–110.

Gieser, D.K. (1992) 'Visual rehabilitation'. *Ophthalmology*, **99**, 1622–1625.

Lancet (1991) 'Retinopathy of prematurity'. **337**, 83–84. *(Editorial.)*

Leat, S.J., Woodhouse, J.M. (1992) 'Reading performance with low vision aids: relationship with contrast sensitivity.' *Ophthalmic and Physiological Optics*, **13**, 9–16.

O'Sullivan, P., Mahoney, G., Robinson, C. (1992) 'Perceptions of pediatricians' helpfulness: a national study of young disabled children.' *Developmental Medicine and Child Neurology*, **34**, 1064–1071.

Quinn, G.E., Dobson, V., Barr, C.C., Davis, B.R., Flynn, J.T., Palmer, E.A., Robertson, J., Trese, M.T. (1991) 'Visual acuity in infants after vitrectomy for severe retinopathy of prematurity.' *Ophthalmology*, **98**, 5–13.

Silverman, W.A. (1980) *Retrolental Fibroplasia: a Modern Parable*. New York: Grune & Stratton.

Sonksen, P., Stiff, B. (1991) *Show Me What My Friends Can See*. London: Institute of Child Health.

Taylor, D. (1990) 'Non-organic disorders.' *In:* Taylor, D. (Ed.) *Pediatric Ophthalmology*. Oxford: Blackwell Scientific, pp. 517–524.

Tresidder, J., Fielder, A.R., Nicholson, J. (1990) 'Delayed visual maturation: ophthalmic and developmental aspects.' *Developmental Medicine and Child Neurology*, **32**, 872–881.

Vernon Committee (1972) *The Education of the Visually Handicapped Child*. London: HMSO.

Walker, E., Tobin, M., McKennell, A. (1992) *Blind and Partially Sighted Children in Britain: the RNIB Survey. Volume 2*. London: HMSO.

8
THE ROLE OF THE PAEDIATRICIAN

Martin C.O. Bax

A child with a significant visual impairment may well have developmental and behavioural problems directly associated with the visual disability, and these in turn may lead to difficulties for the parents in child rearing. Some visually impaired children will have multiple disabilities which exacerbate these problems. Many families who have a child with a visual disability welcome the opportunity to discuss the problem with someone who not only has some understanding of the visual problem itself but who can also see that problem within the context of the child's whole life. In most developed countries the person who, hopefully, can do this will be the paediatrician who specializes in disability. As will be clear from this book, the child who is visually disabled may see a great range of health and educational personnel; the family can be greatly helped if one individual collates all the various reports made on the child and then discusses them with the parents, interpreting where necessary the information that has been collected. This individual (often referred to as the key worker) may not necessarily be the paediatrican (although in the early years often will be) but might be the ophthalmologist or therapist. Nor need the key worker be the same person throughout the childhood years. Indeed, when the child begins school a teacher may well assume this responsibility.

This chapter reviews the task of the paediatrician to whom the visually disabled child is referred, and considers the situation where s/he takes on the role as key worker. The paediatrician's duties in relationship to the visually disabled child can be discussed under the following headings: (i) 'identification; (ii) diagnosis; (iii) assessment; (iv) immediate and long-term management; (v) adolescence; (vi) planning for adult life. In encompassing these tasks the paediatrician will have to look at all aspects of the child's physical health, cognitive and learning abilities and behaviour problems.

Identification
The paediatrician should be concerned to see that a child with significant visual disability is identified as early as possible so that appropriate management, and help for the family, may be instigated.

A number of congenital causes of visual disability, such as anophthalmia or cataract, should be identified on the neonatal ward, and every child's visual function should be reviewed at this time. The examiner should check the visual apparatus itself and observe following. Unfortunately, the examination of neonates is very often carried out by quite junior doctors whose experience of visual problems may be slight. Also, as babies are very often discharged from hospital very rapidly, the infant may never have been in an alert and appropriate state for a functional visual examination to have taken place. Consequently, babies may arrive home without visual function having been assessed. It is therefore enormously important that routine examination by doctors and nurses in the early weeks of life should always include a full visual assessment.

In most countries early assessment is carried out by public health nurses and a doctor (often the general practitioner). The paediatrician has a duty to ensure that whoever is undertaking this task is competent to observe visual function in the young child and, when there is any difficulty achieving this in a particular child, aware enough of the problems to refer that child to the paediatrician.

I do not propose to discuss the normal development of visual function as this is very ably done by Atkinson and Van Hof-van Duin in Chapter 2. However, there are certain situations where identification can be difficult, the most prominent of which is where the child has visual agnosia. In early reports (Illingworth 1961, Mellor and Fielder 1980) it was suggested that these babies eventually did well, but more recently the outlook for their development other than their visual function has been questioned (Fielder *et al.* 1985). Visual agnosia is quite common in children with other disabilities such as cerebral palsy, and in these circumstances assessment can be very difficult. The child with visual agnosia will be referred to the ophthalmologist, who may report that the visual apparatus and pathways are normal and that visual evoked responses are also within the normal range, but they are unable to see normal visual function. In the child who has no other symptomatology, one usually finds that despite the apparent lack of any visual function the child's other development is normal, unlike the blind child who tends to be late in development. The recovery from apparent absent vision to good following and clear evidence of reasonable function at some distance can occur very rapidly.

Case history

A.D. had a stormy perinatal period, being born at 34 weeks gestation, and was first seen in the child development centre at age 6 months (*i.e.* four and a half months from her expected date of delivery). By that time she clearly had cerebral palsy with classic involvement of all four limbs, the lower limbs being worse affected than the upper, but with rigidity as a more prominent sign than spasticity. She was an extremely irritable baby who cried frequently for no apparent reason and was very difficult to feed. There was a disorganized EEG, and occasional possible epileptic phenomena were observed clinically. Monocular movements and roving eye movements were common.

Ophthalmological opinion was that there were no abnormalities and the visual evoked responses were normal. However, neither the ophthalmologist nor the paediatrician observed following, although the mother reported that the child did look at her. Slowly, over the following year, there was a gradual general improvement in her condition and she became much less irritable. Although it was clear she was still occasionally having some minor seizures, the decision was taken not to use anticonvulsants. Her focused eye

110

movements became more and more easily visible, and at 16 months good following, near and far, was observed for the first time, although occasionally—particularly when tired—monocular movements could still be seen. The EEG, although disorganized, showed less seizure activity.

As time goes on the family will naturally be extremely anxious about the child's vision and will want the child to be observed on a regular basis. If the child has some other disability the assessment will be even more difficult.

Diagnosis

While in some instances the diagnosis of the child's visual problem may be purely 'ophthalmic', very often the paediatrician and ophthalmologist will work together in assessing the child's problems. With the 'small' baby, ultrasound and other findings may have suggested that there will be visual problems, and the ophthalmologist and paediatrician will be working together from the beginning. Often genetic, metabolic and further imaging studies will be necessary to confirm the diagnosis.

There are many congenital conditions (see Chapter 4) which feature some degree of visual impairment. The London Neurogenetics Database (Baraitser and Winter 1991) lists a total of 28 syndromes under the mandatory feature blindness (Table 8.1A) and a further 17 which include non-specific visual impairment (Table 8.1B).

Apart from these genetic syndromes, visual impairment is commonly associated with conditions such as cerebral palsy and other neurodevelopmental disorders. In the case cited above, visual problems presented at the same time as the cerebral palsy.

Case history

K.L. was an adopted child. When first seen, aged 4 years, he had retinopathy of prematurity and no useful vision. However, the neonatal period was reported to have been normal, and no particular problems had been noted, although social circumstances meant that the early medical history was rather inadequate. Apart from his visual problems his general development and gross and fine motor functions were normal. His hearing, confirmed by auditory evoked responses, was also normal. His language was delayed, and he used rather telegrammatic speech. He had some stereotypies but these were not very marked, and initially a cautiously optimistic prognosis was given. However, over the next four years it became apparent that he had a broader range of problems: he developed epilepsy; his speech and language remain highly idiosyncratic; he has developed no symbolic play; his social relationships with his adoptive parents were always extremely difficult—he is unable to show affection in a normal way—and now it would be reasonable to diagnose him as a blind, autistic, retarded child.

The problems of paediatric diagnosis of a child with neurological problems have been discussed elsewhere (Aicardi 1992).

TABLE 8.1

Syndromes including blindness or non-specific visual impairment as a feature*

A. Blindness as a feature
AB variant GM2 gangliosidosis, GM2 activator deficiency
Carbonic anhydrase II deficiency (marble brain disease)
Cerebral calcifications and cerebellar hypoplasia
Cerebro–ocular–muscular syndrome (COMS)
Cutis verticis gyrata–mental retardation
Dysosteosclerosis
Fetal vitamin A syndrome
Fryns (1977) – short stature, mental retardation, detached retina
Glycogenosis VII (Tarui), fatal infantile muscle phosphofructokinase deficiency
GMl gangliosidosis infantile form (type I)
Growth retardation–alopecia–pseudoanodontia–optic atrophy (GAPO)
Gyrate atrophy of choroid and retina
Heide (1981) – osteoporosis, blindness, mental retardation
Hernandez (1985) – cortical blindness, polydactyly, mental retardation
Hornova–Dluhosova – primary amyloidosis of gingiva/conjunctiva, mental retardation
Joubert – cerebellar vermis aplasia plus other anomalies
Leber amaurosis
Microcephaly–chorioretinal dysplasia (autosomal dominant)
Mitochondrial myopathy, encephalopathy, lactic acidosis, stroke (MELAS)
Norrie disease
Osteoporosis–pseudoglioma–mental retardation
Phillips (1979) – thoracic dystrophy, retinal aplasia
Rosenberg–Chutorian – optic atrophy, peroneal muscular atrophy, deafness
Spongy degeneration (Canavan), van Bogaert–Bertrand
Temtamy (1974) – metaphyseal dysplasia, anetoderma, optic atrophy
Warfarin embryopathy
Wilkes (1983) – microphthalmia, microcornea, mental retardation
Yolken (1976) – short limbed dwarfism, bowed femurs, irregular metaphyses

B. Non-specific visual impairment as a feature
Benign intracranial hypertension
Colobomas–brachydactyly (type Sorsby)
Creutzfeldt–Jakob
Familial cerebromeningeal angiomatosis (Divry–van Bogaert)
Growth retardation–alopecia–pseudoanodontia–optic atrophy (GAPO)
Hersh (1982) – pigmentary retinopathy, deafness, mental retardation, dysmorphism
Hess (1974) (N-syndrome) – deafness, spasticity, dysmorphic facies
Infantile Refsum
Jarmas (1981) – microcephaly, falciform retinal folds
Keratitis–ichthyosis–deafness syndrome (KID)
Maumenee (1977) – cleft lower lip, chorioretinal degeneration
Ohdo (1986) – mental retardation, congenital hip dysplasia, blepharophimosis, ptosis, hypoplastic teeth
Optic nerve hypoplasia
Refsum disease (hereditary motor and sensory neuropathy type IV)
Sialidosis type II juvenile form (Goldberg)
Spongiform encephalopathy (Gerstmann–Straussler)
Usher – retinitis pigmentosa, deafness

*Adapted by permission from Baraitser and Winter (1991) (references at source).

Assessment

The diagnosis of the child hopefully provides one with information about the underlying disease process and pathology, but it does not give a view of the child's level of function. Even with a severe genetic defect, the consequences will vary with the individual's specific phenotype and the subsequent environmental influences. Every child therefore needs a full functional assessment, and this needs to be repeated at intervals as the course of the pathological process develops, as with case K.L. above. I have described the traditional assessment of the child with developmental problems elsewhere (Bax *et al.* 1990). Essentially, all aspects of the child's development need assessing regularly. These are: gross and fine motor functions, vision, hearing, speech and language, perceptual and intellectual development and, most importantly, social and emotional development. Aspects of all these different functions may be assessed by other professionals; for example, a speech therapist (pathologist) will assess the child's speech and language level. The paediatrician's role is to look at all aspects of the child's development and bring these together. At the same time s/he needs regularly to assess the child's physical status. In terms of development s/he is looking for height, weight and physical growth of the child, including head circumference, and s/he will also observe any physical illness. Assessment looks at specific areas of function, and one of the tasks of the paediatrican is to try to pull all this information together and make a decision about the overall level of the child's development, which can be very difficult. Again, K.L. is a good example of this, the initial assessment having led the paediatrician (me) to think that the child's eventual function might be quite good, whereas continuing assessment proved me wrong and led to the outcome described. It emphasizes an important point about assessment, that it is a process that continues over time, and a period of observation in a nursery setting affords an observation of change. Development over time is an important part of the assessment process.

In general, in terms of fitting the different functions together and thinking about the child's overall outcome, prognosis is obviously easier the later it is undertaken. Indeed, good early motor development is not highly predictive of later intellectual development. The social responses, particularly in the visually disabled child, are an extremely important element in the assessment. The child who rapidly learns her/his social environment—*i.e.* distinguishing parents from grandparents and siblings, and responding to individuals appropriately with affection to those s/he knows and likes and with caution to strangers—even if her/his speech and language development is delayed, has, in my view, a better outlook than the child who is slow at learning social skills.

Nevertheless, assessment of the child's development is often extremely difficult, particularly in relation to language development. A child with vision develops from around age 15 months a rapidly expanding vocabulary: 'car', 'dog', 'drinkie' and 'shoes' are familiar examples of early words. 'Drink' and 'shoes' are relatively easily accessible to the blind child—s/he feels shoes put on, s/he has a drink—but how does s/he understand 'car' or 'dog'? The next stage, which involves expansion of this vocabulary, is even more problematic. 'Car' expands into 'bus', 'truck', 'lorry', 'van', and then to 'Ford', 'Renault', 'BMW'. 'Drink' goes in all sorts of directions: 'cup', 'mug', 'glass', 'bottle' for the object from which the drink comes, and for the drink itself, 'milk', 'orange', 'tea', 'water', etc. These semantic examples must pose great problems for the visually disabled child.

The observer may therefore decide that these difficulties account for the continued delay in the child's language development, and indeed they may. But equally, despite these difficulties, visually disabled children do develop language, albeit later than the normal child, and the clinician's problem is to decide when the language delay cannot be explained by the visual disability alone and to recognize that the child has, in addition to the visual disability, delays in other aspects of development associated with pathology of parts of the CNS other than the visual pathways.

Immediate and long-term management

Too often, although assessment of the child is comprehensive, the paediatrician feels her/his role is not significant because other 'experts' will assist with day-to-day management of the child. In practice, families often have continuing problems which are not related purely to vision and which they will wish to discuss. The developmental problems of the visually impaired child are often perplexing to the parents and equally so to the professional. However, listening to the parents is a useful therapeutic exercise, and discussion will lead both professional and parent to a better understanding of the child's problems.

The dilemma for parents of a disabled child is how far should s/he be treated as a normal child, and to what extent does the disability mean that s/he requires special child rearing? When confronted with a disability, the natural reaction of both parents and professionals is to try to cancel the disability out in some way; for instance, the parent of a child with a motor disability such as cerebral palsy may focus on attempts to improve motor function, neglecting other areas of development. The child with a visual disability presents a different problem. The family and professionals are confronted with the fact that there are no 'exercises' or therapy that can restore missing visual function. Therefore, they try at once to think of ways to achieve what vision gives us in some other way. Indeed, this is appropriate. The developing of other senses to try to take over some aspects of normal visual function is discussed in other chapters in this book. The family want to be given suggestions as soon as they see the disability team.

Case history

I.T., through a chapter of unfortunate circumstances, did not present until age 10 months with bilateral retinoblastomas, for which the eyes had to be enucleated. He was not referred by the ophthalmologist to a developmental team for some time because it was felt that he would develop normally. However, when referred some time over the age of 2 years he was extremely disturbed and overall functioning was well under chronological age. He had no symbolic play, only echolalic speech, and his subsequent outcome was not good. At the initial visit, the parents' main concern was whether there was anything they could do for the child. The inexperienced paediatrician noted that the child would bang with his hands in play and suggested that he should have opportunities for water and sand play. This was initiated and the child very much enjoyed this. A more experienced colleague later pointed out that sand and water was not the best play material for a blind child, as to a large extent they remain abstract, and recommended flour and water, as these substances can be made into shapes and into cakes, and so bring the child in touch with the real world. Nevertheless, initially something for the parents to do had been suggested.

Such strategies should, as far as possible, fit in with the normal daily life of the family, so that any special equipment or toys should be seen as things that the non-disabled child might use albeit in a slightly different way.

As school experience develops, the parents will have access to a range of people who have sophisticated ideas about the processes for helping the child, and the family will want to discuss with the key worker the way that such management is brought into their daily lifestyle.

There are particular points in the life of a disabled child that present almost as crises for the family, and these the disability team should be aware of and plan to meet well in advance. They are diagnosis, schooling, puberty and adolescence, and adult life.

The moment of diagnosis and the problem of telling a family that they have a severely disabled child has been much discussed (see Bax *et al.* 1990). Briefly, the family will often go through a process of mourning for the normal child, and if resolution does not occur the child may be actively or passively rejected. The parents of an anophthalmic child recently refused to take the baby home from hospital and asked that adoption should be arranged (which it was). More difficult for the professional is the family for whom the parents' acceptance of the child is still accompanied by much unresolved anger and grief, and psychiatric help is sometimes useful in these situations.

After the early years the family begin to think of a school placement for the child and this again confronts them with the realities of the disability while the advantages and disadvantages of integration or special school are discussed. Mainstreaming or integrating have been extensively promoted as the best option in recent years, following legislation both in the UK and in the USA. Integration of a severely disabled child is expensive, and in today's economic climate education authorities often pay only lip service to the notion without providing the financial resources to make it a practical reality. The visually disabled child who has additional disabilities may very often be best placed in a well-resourced special school.

Adolescence
Once the solution to the school problem has been achieved, and hopefully it is one

that the parents accept, early school years may go well for both the child and the parents. Ideally, the child will have expectations of doing well and will be reassured by the supportive environment around her/him. It is an unresolved issue as to when a child really understands the extent of the difference between a disabled person and a non-disabled person, but personal experience suggests that it occurs around puberty. Puberty is a biological process in which the physical changes take place that lead to full physical, sexual and *intellectual* maturity. It is worth noting that while the sexual changes are complete between 13 and 15 years of age (earlier for girls than for boys), physical growth and some intellectual development continue after this. There is evidence that the disabled person may actually show an increase in intelligence as late as 20 or 21 years of age, particularly when s/he has had a slow start in life.

Adolescence describes the social changes that in all societies are associated with the passage from childhood to adulthood, and they involve the young person in four interlinked processes: (1) the achievement of self-identity; (2) the achievement of independence; (3) the development of a vocational life activity; and (4) the achievement of adult sexuality. In all these areas the visually disabled person has potential difficulties.

In addition, the parents or carers also may find the process of the young person through these stages more difficult than they would with a normal child. For example, parents of normal children often find it hard to accept their child's emerging sexuality, and this may be particularly difficult for parents of disabled children, who sometimes feel it somehow inappropriate for their son or daughter to have such feelings. Equally, the achievement of independence—doing things on one's own—is particularly worrying for such parents, who may feel that the child's disability makes independence an unrealistic goal. Sometimes this may indeed be the case, but nevertheless the parents have to understand that, even if the young person is going to need some sheltered environment, possibly for life, s/he *must* achieve independence from the family because families by their nature grow old and are not able to sustain the caring process for ever. Therefore, just as the non-disabled young adult moves away and sets up her/his own home, so too must the disabled young adult, whatever the difficulties that this involves.

Planning for adult life

Recent reports have indicated the difficulties experienced by young disabled adults (Beardshaw 1988, Thomas *et al.* 1989). In many countries the services for the multiply disabled young adult are currently very poor, but more and more attention is being focused on the problem. There are many accounts by blind people of their success in adult life, and the young person who is cognitively intact and without additional disability can plan and hopefully expect to achieve adult independence, a vocational job, and a life fully integrated into society. However, in developed countries now a large proportion of visually impaired people have multiple disabilities, and their situation in adult life is more questionable. Very often they

116

will need the continued help of a health, social and educational team to advise them.

Some paediatricians feel that they cannot adequately deal with all the issues involved in the management of a multiply disabled young person, and in some centres departments of adolescent medicine will become involved at the appropriate time. However, many paediatricians who are interested and experienced with disability will try to maintain contact with the disabled young person until s/he reaches adulthood and will hope at that point to be able to organize that the person will have her/his continuing needs met by a suitable adult disability team. Again, individual variation is appropriate, but constant review of the family's problems should be undertaken, including an appraisal of the professionals' effectiveness, and consideration of the need for other expertise in managing the young person's disability.

REFERENCES

Aicardi, J. (1992) *Diseases of the Nervous System in Childhood. Clinics in Developmental Medicine No. 115–118.* London: Mac Keith Press.

Baraitser, M., Winter, R.M. (1991) *London Neurogenetics Database.* Oxford: Oxford University Press.

Bax, M., Hart, H., Jenkins, S.M. (1990) *Child Development and Child Health.* Oxford: Blackwell Scientific.

Beardshaw, V. (1988) *Last on the List: Community Services for People with Physical Disabilities.* London: King's Fund.

Fielder, A.R., Russell-Eggitt, I.R., Dodd, K.L., Mellor, D.H. (1985) 'Delayed visual maturation.' *Transactions of the Ophthalmological Societies of the United Kingdom,* **104**, 653–661.

Illingworth, R.S. (1961) 'Delayed visual maturation.' *Archives of Disease in Childhood,* **36**, 407–409.

Mellor, D.H., Fielder, A.R. (1980) 'Dissociated visual development: electrodiagnostic studies in infants who are "slow to see".' *Developmental Medicine and Child Neurology,* **22**, 327–335.

Thomas, A.P., Bax, M.C.O., Smyth, D.P.L. (1989) *The Health and Social Needs of Young Adults with Physical Disabilities. Clinics in Developmental Medicine No. 106.* London: Mac Keith Press.

9
COMMUNITY BASED PAEDIATRIC MANAGEMENT

Jacqueline Nicholson

This chapter examines the role of community based health services in meeting the needs of children with visual impairments and their families. A community child health service should seek to ensure the good general health and development of all children, thus allowing maximum participation in educational opportunities, the promotion of social and emotional growth within the family, and encouragement of the child's rightful place in adult society. To achieve this, there is a need for early identification and assessment, using multidisciplinary teams. Children of school age and their teachers need support to recognize the limitations imposed by a visual impairment and to meet the special needs that result. Throughout, the role of the community doctor is to help establish and maintain a policy on screening and assessment while ensuring effective communication between all those involved in delivering and receiving services.

In the UK* such teams are usually led by a paediatrician devoting most or all of her/his time to community work; working alongside her/him would be other doctors, clinical medical officers, community based nurses, health visitors and school nurses.

The comparatively small number of significantly visually impaired children within any one health authority area, together with the historical tendency for such children to be educated in specialized teaching facilities (often outside that area), have resulted in limited experience of such children for family practitioners, community nurses and community doctors alike. This lack of experience needs to be addressed when attempting to provide appropriate services.

During the 1980s a shift in attitudes and practice occurred which resulted in the visually impaired child being more likely to be educated within the area of her/his local education authority and, indeed, within a local school. This principle is now enshrined within the legislation of many countries, for example the 1981 Education Act in England and Wales. It is therefore vital that community child health services should be both available and accessible to the child, and that staff are appropriately trained to deliver an acceptable spectrum of support.

---

*This chapter is written within the context of the author's experience of working in community health services within the UK. The principles apply universally, although in other countries the terminology may be different.

Such provision involves coordination and cooperation between the statutory providers of health, education and social services, together with input from voluntary agencies.

In order to ensure that community child health services are able to activate any support mechanisms, it is essential that the service is notified as soon as possible of new cases of visual impairment. Established pathways of communication between hospital and community services are vital, and incorporate the philosophy of an 'integrated child health service'.

Community child health units collate information on children within the local authority and increasingly maintain computerized special needs data bases, including information on children with visual impairments. For this to work it is essential that copies of letters are sent to general practitioners and to the community child health units from the hospital departments where children attend for outpatient or inpatient consultations. This will ensure that community doctors and nurses are kept informed of illness and disability, and enable computer based information to be updated, including special needs registers. This practice is further encouraged, in England and Wales, by recent legislation under the 1989 Children Act, which places a responsibility on health services to work closely with social service departments in the recognition and assessment of disability in children. The Act also requires social service departments to maintain a disability register.

From a central point, information can be transferred to local child health teams, who can offer review and follow-up within the community. A named senior doctor (increasingly a consultant community paediatrician) should have responsibility for management and development of the service.

The community paediatrician has a part to play in both planning and managing services to this group of children as a whole, as well as providing support to the individual child. It would be useful to look at community based services under two headings: responsibility to the professional group and responsibility to the individual and family.

Responsibility to the professional group
Identification of visual impairment
As so much of early development and childhood experience is dependent on the development of vision and the integrity of visual pathways, it is essential that vision problems are detected at the earliest opportunity. Screening is increasingly undertaken by the primary health care team of general practitioner and health visitor.

Screening procedures should be aimed at detecting (i) serious defects, *e.g.* congenital abnormalities such as cataracts or optic atrophy, which can result in partial sightedness or blindness, and (ii) less serious conditions, *e.g.* refractive error and squint. Screening programmes should be accompanied by a programme which highlights 'at risk' groups for which additional procedures should be available, for example examination of preterm babies for retinopathy of prematurity. Screening for associated vision problems in children with other disabling conditions should also be available, such as annual acuity checks in children with Down syndrome who have a higher incidence of myopia. A report by Hall (1989) has outlined an appropriate screening programme in the preschool years. This includes:

- Taking a careful family history, and antenatal and birth histories, which may highlight 'at risk' groups.
- Examination of the eyes in the neonate. Using a +3 lens at a distance of 15–25cm a cataract may be detected as a silhouette against the red reflex. If there is doubt about the result of this examination it should be repeated in six weeks.
- At the 6 week examination, notes to be taken of early visual development, fixation of small objects, following of moving objects, and looking at the carer's face directly.
- The provision of guidelines for parents on the development of vision and common vision problems—a useful education tool.
- At each screening contact within a preschool programme, parents should always be asked about concerns regarding vision.
- Appropriate staff training on normal development of vision would ensure recognition of signs and symptoms of abnormality, *e.g.* abnormal eye movements, poor visual following, etc.
- A recognized referral pathway to specialist opinion and assessment for those failing screening procedures.

The phenomenon of delayed visual maturation should be recognized by health visitors, doctors and community nurses carrying out these examinations. It is imperative to listen to the parents and to follow up any concerns regarding poor use of vision.

The screening of young children for visual problems is fraught with difficulties and has been much discussed (Stewart-Brown 1987, Stewart-Brown *et al.* 1988). There is a case to be made for screening vision at around 3½ years, provided that this is carried out by appropriately trained professionals, *e.g.* an orthoptist (a paramedic concerned with assessment and treatment) working with an optometrist. Routine vision screening continues to be carried out by community based services at school entry and at two to three year intervals throughout school life.

The physical and intellectual development of 'under-5s' is routinely screened, although there is a changing emphasis from screening to the wider aspects of surveillance. Training for child health screening and surveillance lies largely with the community based health services, and proper emphasis should be given to vision during such training programmes.

Statutory responsibilities to education
In England and Wales, under the 1981 Education Act the procedure for assessment of a child lays down statutory responsibilities for each of the agencies. The medical information is usually provided by the locally based clinical medical officer in consultation with other medical and paramedical professionals.

120

Under the terms of this Act there will be a small number of children with a 'significant visual impairment' who will need to have a 'Statement of Educational Needs' completed. There is no agreed definition of a significant visual impairment, and this does not depend on registration of partial sight or blindness. A good working definition is 'a visual impairment such that the child is unable fully to participate and benefit from normal curricular activities in school without additional specialized help'.

In addition to contributing to the initial statement, there is a requirement to review each statemented child on an annual basis. There is a further 'reassessment of needs' at around 14 years of age, with particular reference to potential school leaving issues.

Many regional health authorities have recommended the setting up of special needs registers in each district. This will provide important demographic and statistical information to assist in appropriate planning of services—increasingly essential in times of limited resources. The 1989 Children Act requires social service authorities to establish a register of 'disabled' children, and it is likely that district health authorities will be asked to participate in the identification of such children, possibly using information from a special needs register. The inclusion of visually impaired children on this register will be the community doctor's responsibility.

Inter-agency liaison
Support for visually impaired children and their families comes from many sources, including health, education and social services and voluntary organizations, resulting in planning and management responsibilities for the community paediatrician. Some of the medical support may be 'two centre' based, as a number of children supported locally are also treated and reviewed at specialist regional or national centres.

Inter-agency planning is essential in order to maximize limited resources, capitalize specialist training and prevent unnecessary duplication of services. Success is dependent on good communication, but the size of the potential network of support can defeat that objective. Because much of the service provision lies within the community, it often falls to the community paediatrician to provide essential liaison between services. The appointment within each health authority of a community doctor with special responsibility for the visually impaired child would greatly enhance the likely success of achieving that liaison. In addition, the establishment of a multidisciplinary forum with responsibility for visual impairment has been shown to be a successful medium for identifying gaps in service provision and for furthering the development of communication networks.

Responsibility to the individual
There are four critical periods for a family with a child who has a disability: (i) at diagnosis and assessment; (ii) at primary (junior) school entry (in the UK, at age 5

years); (iii) at secondary school entry (UK, age 11 years); (iv) at school leaving (UK, 16–18 years). In this section the needs at each of these stages will be identified, along with the criteria for service provision. Specific examples from the UK system are used to illustrate the recommendations.

Diagnosis and assessment

The diagnosis of significant visual impairment is the start of an often confusing journey for child and parents through a maze of professionals, all seemingly with a justified interest and input. They may move from the community developmental screening unit to an ophthalmologist, then to a paediatrician, perhaps to a neurologist, to a child development centre and then back to the community doctor, contacting *en route* the education and social services!

The community paediatrician can be a vital bridge between primary, secondary and tertiary health care levels, in addition to maintaining links with the local education and social service departments.

Diagnosis is usually made by the ophthalmologist who has the responsibility to communicate back to both the primary health care team and community child health services, and to ensure appropriate hospital follow-up and referral.

All children with significant visual impairment should be fully assessed by a paediatric team. This assessment will identify associated medical problems, clarify general development, and provide opportunities for genetic counselling and screening of hearing. Within such an assessment a formidable list of professionals, including ophthalmologist, orthoptist, optometrist, paediatrician, geneticist, audio-metrist, educational psychologist, speech therapist, social worker, advisory teacher, mobility officer, physiotherapist and occupational therapist, may all become involved. A community paediatrician may also be included: her/his role includes coordinating information, and feedback to the family, the health visitor, the general practitioner and other community services. The community doctor is in the unique position of translating the strengths and weaknesses of the child to the direct situation in which that child has to live and function.

Following identification of a visual problem and assessment, there should be feedback to the community child health team—particularly important if a community paediatrician is not included in the assessment team. Such notification should trigger the community child health team into providing follow-up in conjunction with hospital services. If the community doctor has not already been involved, an invitation to see the child either in clinic or at home should be extended. Home visits are particularly valuable to families who are often overwhelmed by the practical problems of travel, maintaining hospital appoint-ments, and coping with the emotional and psychological cost of coming to terms with a child who may be blind.

Many of the recommendations from a team meeting will involve community based services—health visitor support, advisory teacher support and social service input. The community paediatrician is in a unique position to ensure that such recommendations are carried out. A follow-up appointment may also be made to ensure recommendations are in place, and a six-monthly review in the local clinic or nursery ensures some continuity in support. This is particularly important for a family who may be receiving support from two centres.

Children who have rare conditions are frequently reviewed both locally and at tertiary centres of excellence. This may involve the family in a disproportionate amount of travelling, having to cope with two teams and the different ways in which the same information can be communicated. The additional stress that this can place on a family should not be underestimated. Families struggling to come to terms with lifelong disability find hospital environments threatening, and they may omit to ask the very questions that concern them most. An informed, accessible community doctor can be a valuable source of contact and reassurance, sometimes acting as an advocate for the parent and child. There is an important role in ensuring that professional information is communicated between two centres.

There is also a part to play in reinforcing the existence and role of voluntary organizations. While parents will be informed of such organizations during the assessment procedure, there is frequently a block to this additional information as the family are still coming to terms with the diagnosis and its long term implications. There is thus a need to reiterate information at a later date when the family are emotionally more prepared to be identified with the visually impaired group, and therefore to find the link acceptable.

The diagnosis of long term visual impairment is a body blow to parents, and there is a vital need to cushion this as much as possible. There should be recognition that the diagnosis is akin to a bereavement for many parents. They will go through many of the emotional and psychological stages of bereavement, disbelief, guilt and anger. They and the extended family need support and counselling, and this is an additional role for the community doctor, who from the clinic base may be more accessible than the hospital department.

An information pack for families of newly diagnosed blind or partially sighted children should be available. Such a pack should be the result of close cooperation between all the professional agencies and local voluntary organizations. The community paediatrican will have a role to play in this and indeed could be the instigator of such a development. This would complement the leaflets produced by a number of national organizations (*e.g.* Royal National Institute for the Blind in the UK, American Foundation for the Blind, Canadian Institute for the Blind) by giving information on specific local services and procedures.

School entry

By the time the visually impaired child reaches school age there may have been a shift in the monitoring of health care. If the visual impairment is of a non-progressive nature, and if the child has no other ongoing medical problems, input from the consultant paediatrician and child development centre may be greatly reduced. Indeed, the child may have been discharged from some departments. In such cases, the community child health doctor, ophthalmologist and general practitioner will provide the monitoring role.

Significant visual impairment can lead to learning difficulties, language delay and problems with social integration and communication in its widest sense. Ultimately there will be possible restrictions to career opportuniies. To meet these special needs, visually impaired children have been educated in special schools, many of them residential, or in special units attached to mainstream schools. More recently, a policy of integration has increased the number of children in mainstream schools supported by a resource facility.

The community doctor's role in the school is both individual and corporate. There is a responsibility to the child and her/his parents, but also to teachers and professional carers within the school, to ensure the success of the child's placement.

Before the child enters school it is essential that the ground be properly prepared. If there has been ongoing contact between the community paediatrician and the child and parents, there will have been opportunities for educational implications of the vision problem to have been discussed. Increasingly children with vision impairment are offered nursery placements, and with the educational shift toward integration many children will have been in a mainstream nursery at least on a part-time basis. The community paediatrician will be involved in the statutory processes leading to educational placement, such as the statutory assessment in England and Wales under the 1981 Education Act. The provision of a medical report collating relevant information for the education authority has already been mentioned.

Once placement has commenced, the child should be offered a six-monthly review by the designated community child health doctor to the nursery. Working with and reasssuring teaching staff who may have little or no knowledge of visual disability is an important role. Parents also need to be reassured that their child will enjoy the school experience. The school doctor should be available to parents and teachers alike to answer queries, share anxieties and address difficulties. Although an annual review is all that is statutorily required, at least termly assessment of the situation should be offered in the initial stages of education. It may not be necessary to have 'hands on' contact with the child on a termly basis, but regular contact with the school and feedback to parents is essential. This policy should be adhered to when the child moves from nursery to infant school. There are numerous issues which need to be addressed.

THE PHYSICAL ENVIRONMENT

The sight restrictions of the visually impaired child may have led to delay in gross motor development, some possible abnormalities in freedom of movement, bad posture, low self-esteem, lack of confidence in freely moving in a new environment, and a greatly reduced visual experience. These need to be taken into consideration when planning the physical environment in which the child is to play and work in nursery and school, to ensure that the child can function maximally and develop her/his full potential. Attention needs to be given to lighting, possible visual distractions, layout of classrooms, the use of, and the contrast of, teaching materials within the classroom, and the appropriateness of posters and other decorations.

The safety of the physical environment is of paramount importance. Access to and from the building, the nature of floor surfaces in both playground and classroom, the safety of stairs with respect to highlighting stair edges, stair surfaces and the provision of safety rails, the provision of clear visual markers in the playground to prevent disorientation, the nature of play equipment in the playground, and the ability to move independently in and out of the classrooms all need to be considered.

SOCIAL INTEGRATION

Severely visually impaired children will have been at a grave disadvantage prior to moving into school. Learning opportunities will have been reduced, and this is particularly true of social learning. Blind children are not aware of 'body language', may have developed stereotypic play behaviour, and will have some limitations to language development, particularly with respect to comprehension of conceptual situations. All of these factors may mitigate against the child being successfully integrated into a peer group. Awareness of this likelihood is essential, and teachers and parents should be appropriately prepared for an initially anxious transition period as the child moves from home to the school situation.

SELF-HELP SKILLS

As well as the social dependence that many children with a sensory impairment may have, there is often a delay in the development of self-help skills. For instance, dressing and undressing may be delayed in the visually impaired child. The development of normal eating habits is often delayed or distorted. Weaning may have been very difficult to establish, and the introduction of new tastes and textures may frequently have been problematic. Young children, particularly moving into a nursery situation, may still have very specific feeding habits and requirements which need to be understood and allowed for.

GENERAL HEALTH

It is important to ensure that school staff are aware of any associated medical problems, including hearing status. However, it is more usual for a visually impaired child to be in all other respects normal and healthy, and this fact should be stressed so that the visual disability is seen in context.

The school doctor should be readily available for consultation with both parents and school during the initial introduction to school life. Many school authorities hold regular termly meetings of special needs children with educational psychologists, school staff, visiting teacher services and the school doctor, and these provide a useful forum for updating and addressing areas of concern. These consultations should include a review of the visual problem, any associated medical problems, and a check on hearing. There should be an opportunity for updating on the child's academic progress, particularly with respect to literacy and numeracy skills.

As visually impaired babies frequently have feeding problems, and often resist attempts at oral hygiene, it is important to check dental health.

Assessment of mobility and physical independence is an essential part of every review. Visually impaired children are frequently very restricted in their independence opportunities, and may be overprotected by naturally anxious parents. They are, therefore, more likely to be socially isolated, particularly at weekends and in school holidays. They do not develop the 'streetwiseness' of their peer group. Within the confines of home or school they can appear positive and outgoing, but when removed to a new environment, particularly the High Street, can become apprehensive and fearful. Mobility training should be offered to all children with a significant visual impairment. Some education authorities fund mobility officer posts specifically to support preschool children and children in school. However, in practice resources are usually very stretched and many authorities can offer only a limited service to children in this respect.

The older schoolchild

At least a year before leaving junior school, plans should be made for the transfer to secondary education. Parents should be made aware of the options available at secondary school level, and together with the child have an opportunity to visit secondary establishments. Once again the school doctor will have a role, with professional colleagues, in ensuring that the child's requirements with respect to physical environment, safety aspects, social integration and development of independence are all addressed in the transfer.

Secondary education brings its own challenges. The nature of secondary education is fundamentally different to that of the primary school. The secondary school is invariably bigger both geographically and numerically. The design of the curriculum means that there is more movement within the building from one department to another. The content of the curriculum will expose the visually impaired child to additional challenges and possible hazards, for example in the science laboratory. The volume of work to be completed within unit time is increased, and there is a greater stress placed on independent individual work.

It is vital that all these issues are addressed prior to transfer and are understood by the child, parents and staff. This provides additional challenge in that the size of the staff roll may be at least ten times that of the primary school; it is important that every member of staff who may come into contact with the visually impaired child is aware of the issues relating to that child's successful integration both educationally and socially. Inclusion in the staff roll of a designated member of staff responsible for special needs ('special needs coordinator') greatly facilitates successful communication, and there should be regular opportunities for the doctor to meet with the coordinator to address staff anxieties.

During the annual review particular attention should be paid to the social integration of the child, with respect to both school and home life. Adolescence is often a stressful and ill-understood period for many young people and their families, and the additional burden of coping with a disability which is frequently resented and rejected by the child at this time requires sensitivity, understanding and support. Many young people with disabling conditions who have coped very well in primary school find the challenges of integration at secondary school fraught with difficulties and disappointment. Young people and their families should know that they have regular opportunities to discuss these issues with the school doctor.

During the secondary school period, the community doctor may be asked to submit a report to public examination bodies on behalf of the pupil, supporting a request for special examination arrangements in the light of the disabling condition.

School leaving

At this stage the visually impaired child has moved into adolescence and is approaching adulthood. The confusing status of adolescence, together with anxieties about self-confidence, coping abilities and peer group acceptance are compounded with new anxieties regarding career prospects. The young person at this stage will move from the relatively protected and supported world of school to the often threatening and far less protected world of the workplace.

An increasing number of adolescents will move into further education, but most of the statutory provisions do not extend beyond school leaving. Some education authorities provide advisory teachers for sight impaired students to work in post-school placements such as colleges of further education, and this is a valuable adjunct where in place.

A school leaver's case conference at the beginning of the last year at school will provide an opportunity for the school doctor to liaise with teachers, the careers service, colleges of further education, community education workers, youth workers and possible employers, and should be an essential part of preparation for the workplace. The conference should aim to ensure that all ongoing health needs of the young person will be met by adult health services, including follow-up by the ophthalmology department and by the appropriate physician if there are associated health problems, and that the general practitioner is aware of the school leaving situation and the next placement. The doctor should also ensure that adult paramedical services will continue to provide, for example, speech therapy and physiotherapy, and that the school-leaver and her/his family are aware of appropriate national and local voluntary organizations and agencies. Opportunities for genetic counselling for the young person should be considered and offered.

It may be helpful to nominate a key worker who will maintain links with the young person and her/his family for the initial 12 months after leaving school. This would not normally be the role of the school doctor, as community child health services are not offered beyond school leaving age. The school doctor should, however, ensure that a summary report of the school leaver's case conference is sent to the family doctor and to all health professionals who will continue to provide support.

In addition, the production of an information booklet for 'special needs' school leavers has been found beneficial by those authorities which have pioneered their use, and community child health services can have an important role to play in both promoting and contributing to such information.

The careers service has the most important role to play in this particular transition phase for the visually impaired young person. Employment opportunities are particularly difficult for all young persons with a disability, and detailed assessment of needs and skills, and counselling with respect to career choices, is vital. The school doctor will have a responsibility to ensure that the careers service is fully aware of relevant medical and health issues that may influence the successful choices of employment.

Recommendations

1. Appointment of a designated doctor within the community child health services with responsibility for visual impairment, to develop services, review screening and assessment procedures, and undertake responsibility for supporting children in local education authority facilities.

2. The establishment of a protocol for vision screening as part of a core programme of developmental screening and assessment within community child health services.

3. The establishment of a policy following the diagnosis of significant visual impairment. This should be agreed with ophthalmologists, paediatricians, community child health services, and education and social services.

4. The provision of adequate staff training in all aspects of visual development.

5. The targeting of some staff for additional training in the management of visual impairment.

6. The development of an information pack for families of visually impaired children (a multi-agency initiative).

7. The establishment of good medical communication pathways between community paediatric services, ophthalmologists and hospital paediatric services. The practice of sending copy letters from hospital paediatricians and ophthalmology departments to community child health services greatly facilitates this communication, and will ensure that community doctors are aware of children with visual impairment.

8. The establishment of a referral pathway to advisory teachers and social services. This is essential to ensure preschool input and immediate post-diagnostic support.

9. The establishment of a multidisciplinary forum to review service provision on a regular basis.

10. The establishment of regular multi-agency professional meetings in education establishments with a visually disabled pupil on roll.

11. Involvement in, and encouragement of, locally based parent support groups.

12. A commitment to continue to care.

REFERENCES

Hall, D.M.B. (1989) *Health for All Children. A Programme for Child Health Surveillance.* Oxford: Oxford University Press.

Stewart-Brown, S. (1987) 'Visual defects in school children: screening policy and educational implications.' *In:* MacFarlane, J.A. (Ed.) *Progress in Child Health, Vol. 3.* Edinburgh: Churchill Livingstone, pp. 14–37.

—— Haslum, M.N., Howlett, B. (1988) 'Pre-school vision screening, a service in need of rationalisation.' *Archives of Disease in Childhood*, **63**, 356–359.

10
PLANNING A PROGRAMME FOR THE MULTIPLY DISABLED CHILD

Janet Edwards

The following description of a method of programme planning for the multiply disabled, visually impaired child is based on that employed at Woodcroft School, Loughton, Essex, UK, an independent day school which, like many other schools in other settings throughout the world, has developed its own individual approach. This approach has evolved out of many years experience with such children, their parents, physicians, teachers and therapists, and through studies in hospitals, schools and other centres. It has also been influenced by the several publications gathered in the bibliography at the end of this chapter.

The school, which has been providing a comprehensive service for over 30 years, is situated to the north-east of London in Epping Forest. With an intake from a number of Education Authorities in the London area and neighbouring rural counties, there is a balance of socio-economic and cultural backgrounds among the pupils. The Special School has 18 places for boys and girls in the 2 to 13 year age range who have varying and multiple special needs, including children also having some degree of visual impairment. It is divided into three classes. There is an adjoining Nursery School for children aged 3 to 5 years who are developing normally, with whom children from the special needs classes integrate.

Each child's day is carefully planned in order to make the most of her/his own potential within the framework of individual development programmes, group work and integrative activities.

Planning takes place at every stage of the child's placement: on a formal basis, for example on entry, at the six week initial assessment described below, and at progress meetings; and informally at daily staff meetings before school starts and at weekly programme planning meetings. As a result, a range of relevant and interested people are able to contribute at some stage to the pupil's ongoing assessment. These people may include parents, teachers, nurses and therapists, and outside specialists such as paediatricians, audiologists, ophthalmologists and other health professionals.

It has been our experience that a programme, planned to encourage the child's growth in confidence and a sense of security within which some development can be achieved during an assessment period of not less than two years, succeeds best with the advice of a visiting paediatrician coming to the school and into the home to relate to the parents and see the child functioning in her/his own environment.

It has also been our experience that underlying physical impairments more often than not affect overall development and that early referral for suitable investigation is essential in order to plan a developmental programme and approach its implementation realistically and efficiently. Paediatric guidance is needed in achieving suitable referral.

Over the years the school has found that successfully planning a programme for the child involves recognizing the point at which s/he is *ready* to receive therapeutic or educational intervention. This readiness is assumed to be when s/he is observably *interested* in the strategies to be tried and giving *assent* to the particular activity on offer.

This belief, that recognizing when a child is ready requires observation, and the fact that observation, if it is to be of value, depends upon a respect for accuracy, has dictated a planned approach, both to assessment and to developing a system which will encourage a realistic and effective means of assisting the child not only to develop, but to do so in ways which allow some satisfaction and fulfilment. The importance of individual and carefully planned developmental programmes has been recognized and applied by maintaining high staff–pupil ratios (one to one for much of the day), by ensuring open and accessible lines of communication between interested parties, and by providing a calm and positive atmosphere in which to nurture the child as s/he matures and grows.

Aims of the programme
In addition to their special needs, we assume that multiply disabled visually impaired children have the same needs as other children. Each pupil, whatever her/his needs, comes to us with abilities and achievements that can form a foundation on which to build, through teaching and therapy, in a school environment. The programme is looked at as a means of addressing each of these children's unique combination of needs and circumstances.

Elements of the programme
Before interview
Before programme planning begins: (i) parents will have visited the school, sometimes with an educational or medical adviser; (ii) the sending authority, usually the education department, with the guidance of the child's paediatrician, the community paediatrician or the school medical officer, will have recommended and agreed to the child being interviewed with her/his parents with a view to a possible placement at the school; and (iii) a home visit by the school's occupational therapist, speech–language therapist or physiotherapist will have been made.

Interview and entry
It is at the interview and entry stage that the programme planning begins. After one interview session, the child enters the school in a manner agreed to be appropriate by parents and others concerned. Thus, if s/he has not left home before,

a parent may attend until it is felt that s/he can manage without their constant presence, and until the one-to-one relationship the school offers every child is seen to have begun to be established. If s/he is transferring from another school, the initial relationship will have been started by visits to and from that school, and the cooperation of previous staff working with the child will be sought in achieving a satisfactory start.

Given information
Certain information on the child is likely to be available at the outset:
• the parents' first-hand description of their child's history to date and their wishes in approaching her/his developing educational needs and treatment;
• a draft or substantive statement of special educational needs (although a child can enter this school while such a statement is being drawn up);
• other medical, psychological and social reports;
• reports from previous schools, clinics or other centres; and
• a note of the child's appearance and observed behaviour and state during a half day interview, including her/his response to people other than parents and to the school environment.

Initial stage
After the first six weeks a programme planning meeting takes place with parents, educational psychologist, paediatrician and all staff concerned, as well as any teacher or other outside adviser already involved in the child's progress. At this meeting the information gathered during the six weeks observation period is presented in note form.

From admission, some initial assessment may be possible to help in deciding realistic day to day goals.

Parents are encouraged to communicate their views, in addition to those wishes expressed and noted before and at interview, by means of the daily home/school diary, by telephone and by visits (parents to school or staff to home). Only domiciliary trained staff undertake home visits.

Observation
Each child is placed in the close overall care of a teacher and in the direct care of a suitable assistant at all times. Based on what is already known of the child, the teacher and assistant will have been carefully chosen. They will need to be capable of relating to the child sympathetically, watching and listening to her/him, and recognizing and accepting her/his feelings and needs. They will also need to have suitable training, experience and skills to be able to encourage and guide her/him and to know when to intervene by offering opportunities for further development, while always keeping her/him open and accessible to other educational and therapeutic strategies. From admission they will commence constant observation, as will all the therapy, curricular and nursing staff (*viz.* music therapist,

occupational therapist*, physiotherapist*, play therapist, speech therapist*, clinical psychologist, English teacher, language teacher, maths teacher, physical education instructor, nursery nurses, medical nurses, psychiatric nurses).

It is our policy to include parents if they so wish in classroom and other activities once the child has been introduced to the new setting. The six weeks to the first planning meeting are considered to be this introductory period, and after this parents are able to come and go freely by arrangement.

Referrals for medical investigations will not usually be made by therapists until the planning meeting; however, such referrals, if thought to be urgent, may be suggested and discussed at home or in school with parents; and during the first six weeks the general practitioner's or other medical opinion may possibly be sought.

Induction

From the moment of entering the school building as a pupil, care is taken to give the child a sense of security through the understanding of her/his assigned teacher and assistant and the space initially given to her/him. At first the classroom, its adjacent bathroom and cloakroom, and specific parts of the school garden are the only places made available to the child. Once s/he has a thorough knowledge of these areas they serve as a base from which s/he can explore the school and its surroundings further, and later launch into the regular weekly afternoon outings from school to the swimming pool, gymnasium, adventure playground, pony riding centre and sports hall, which are gradually offered as appropriate.

Following the child's lead

Based on all the information gathered in the foregoing ways, and taking the lead from the child's approach to what is on offer, options are kept open so that the most suitable setting within the school can be found to suit her/his needs as assessed. S/he is given a free reign, within broad but defined limits with respect to safety and simple social conformity. Any behaviour within these limits is accepted at this stage so that what s/he does can be observed and so that s/he may later be more receptive to suggestions from teachers and therapy staff.

Most teaching and therapeutic intervention proceeds on a one-to-one basis throughout the school, including during class and group work. The availability of a personal assistant is usually retained at least until the planning meeting, and in any case until it is considered that the child no longer needs such constant attention. While this need can be expected to diminish and pass as the child becomes more confident and familiar with other staff and gains in emotional independence, such a major step as weaning her/him from the assistant is taken only in consultation with all concerned, with careful planning to maintain the child's confidence and progress, and with no time limit imposed.

Thought is given to the child's need to know who is with her/him, so that, for

---

*A further home visit is made by at least one of these staff before the first planning meeting.

instance, at staff change-over times care is taken to say what is going on, to introduce the newcomer and to get the child to touch the newcomer's hand or shoulder.

The environment, both indoors and out, is carefully planned to use the senses of touch, hearing, taste and smell as guides and indicators of place, and to help a child learn to move about freely and independently and to be interested and stimulated into curiosity and pleasure in the surroundings. For instance, bathrooms are comfortable and have sound stimuli and pleasant surfaces and smell; tactile trails are on the walls leading from room to room, and certain areas are defined by different floor materials; care is taken to preserve access to major apparatus, *e.g.* rocking horse, sand-tray, etc.; and favourite objects and toys are always kept in the same places. When it is necessary to move a non-ambulant blind child from one place to another, however swiftly and whether in or outdoors, care is taken that s/he is held or wheeled facing the way s/he is going so that s/he can experience stimuli in proper sequence and learn to orientate correctly, *e.g.* feeling the wind on turning the corner of a building and smelling food on entering a kitchen.

Gradually, the child is introduced to the fringes of the small mixed group of not more than six children with whom s/he is likely to mix at times and to integrate at a later date.

Formulating an overall programme
The overall programme for multiply disabled visually impaired children follows the same basic pattern as for all the children in the school. At the first planning meeting with the parents, class teacher, curricular and therapy staff and outside advisers, and with the observations of all other school staff concerned, the occupational therapist presents the child's strengths and needs in the form of typed lists headed: 'Strengths', 'Needs', 'Goals', and 'Adult tasks'. These, with the information now available, form the basis of a programme which allows (i) a child's strengths to be the basis on which a reasonable set of teaching and therapy goals and aims can be built, and (ii) a system of areas of development to be defined and assessed, upon which achievement can be encouraged.

The areas of potential development addressed are: (i) independence skills, (ii) communication skills, (iii) physical skills, (iv) relationships, (v) self expression, and (vi) emotional development. Loosely based on the original Gunzburg Progress Assessment Chart (Gunzburg 1973), these are the broad areas on which the child's programme is built. They also inform the school week: on Mondays to Thursdays the first four are focused on in turn, Friday being set aside as a day for consolidation and project work; all activities give opportunities for self expression and emotional development.

The programme is constantly monitored and reassessed at regular intervals. It will be typed up as a whole and also put into simple diagrammatic form, and circulated to parents and others concerned. For use and guidance in the classroom the programme will also be simplified to step-by-step goals, clearly displayed in a

TABLE 10.1

Elements of the school curriculum

Personal development, including psychological supervision
    (video record)
Language stimulation
Religious education
Creative/expressive, including music and movement, drama
English (national curriculum*)
Mathematics (national curriculum*)
Science (national curriculum*)
Technology (national curriculum*)
Computer and video
Physical education: trampolining, adventure playground,
    gymnasium, pony riding, swimming
Occupational therapy
Speech therapy
Physiotherapy
Music therapy
Nursery/mainstream integration**

*The national curriculum is a statutory system introduced in
the 1988 Education Reform Act to standardize educational
provision in England and Wales.
**See text.

form which can be changed daily.

Each area is given due emphasis in record keeping, an important part of which is a personal video record, with a structured pattern based on the above areas of potential development, which is kept from school entry throughout the child's stay and which is then available to the family and, with parental permission, as a monitoring, teaching, medical and therapy reference to others concerned. In addition, easily maintained programme records are kept which are designed to be readily accessible to everyone, including the child where appropriate.

School curriculum

The child's school curriculum, detailed in Table 10.1, runs alongside the programme, and its components are explored and guided by the child's individual programme requirements, level of ability and needs as assessed. Access to this curriculum is suitably gradual, although most parts of it will be offered and instigated by the end of the first year. It offers a broad spectrum of experience for the child, through a wide selection of staff with whom to relate and of environments to explore and places to visit.

Delivery of the programme

Delivery of the programme in school will be by the multidisciplinary team, with the parents' support and guidance as to the direction and effectiveness of the work, and with their involvement in such practice and consolidation at home and in school as may be appropriate and practical. In school every morning a meeting is held before the children arrive to discuss and plan the day's programme. Weekly programme meetings are also held so that all staff can be involved in planning, monitoring and evaluating their work. In addition to the regular annual reviews, meetings can quickly be arranged by request of parents or staff, these usually taking the form of informal working lunches.

Home visits in term and holiday time are undertaken by therapy staff to discuss progress and to plan the next step as the programme goes from stage to stage. Parents will visit the school to observe, advise and work with teachers and therapy staff.

The child's programme is worked out on a day-to-day basis which allows for:
- individual teaching and therapy;
- group work, including creative/expressive work, therapy and project work;
- social activities, meals, registration, play, classroom routines, outings;
- regular afternoon outings for sporting activities (see above) or to places of interest associated with project work, etc.;
- integration with pupils from mainstream schools at all levels (see below);
- staff evaluation of the programme and monitoring of the child's progress.

Integration

Integration, educationally and socially, with non-disabled children is planned into every child's programme. This is always given careful thought in relation to each child's needs, and readiness and preparation are among the important factors considered. There is regular nursery provision within the school, with two classes of 3- to 5-year-olds; there are three primary schools (ages 5 to 11 years) locally with which we have worked a scheme of part-time integration for many years; three secondary schools (ages 11 to 18 years) which are also able to offer special arrangements to integrate individuals and small groups and which also send pupils into our school to entertain and socialize with the children; and a special school for pupils with moderate and severe learning difficulties with which we work closely. In addition, where appropriate we may suggest to parents that the child be involved from home with local activities such as swimming and sports clubs, the scouting movement and other organizations offering social and physical activities.

Integration takes place in both directions, and non-disabled children of all ages come into the school to share facilities and work in conversation and language groups or to play under proper supervision. They are allocated a skilled teacher/nurse/therapist for as long as such a companion is needed, through whom the demands of the group can be interpreted. On visits to other schools appropriate staff from the special school are always provided to support the child and the host class teacher.

Planned integration on a programmed basis is seen as a means of safely and gradually familiarizing pupils with the variety, stimulation and demands of children's normal activities and interests. It is never undertaken without preparation, and a suitable peer group is chosen with care and discussion with all concerned.

Transfer to next school
Part of the programme is to recognize the signs that the child has outgrown her/his need of this school and is ready to transfer to the next setting, and this is discussed regularly with parents and staff and with the sending authority and other outside advisers, usually after a minimum of two years.

Case study
The development of a programme for one multiply disabled blind child is detailed here to exemplify the planning process.

History and description
Tom entered Woodcroft School at the age of 8 years after a three year preparatory period at a school for blind children. In addition to his blindness he exhibited autistic features, speech and language delay and behavioural disturbance, and at the time of transfer he had recently begun to experience what his adoptive mother termed 'fits'. Although hampered by communication problems he had made useful relationships with at least two members of staff at his previous school and he transferred at its customary top age.

Tom was born in the provinces, adopted at the age of 4 years after a history of going from one foster home to another from birth, and brought to live near London. He was the only child of his adoptive parents. At adoption he was described as 'a blind toddler with only a glimmer of observable awareness of other people', and his original social worker is quoted as never having seen him smile in his first four years. His mother says he was 'tiny and underweight, looked seriously neglected, and though he could walk, he did not.' She remembers him as 'a curled up hedgehog, withdrawn from the world', who took months to show any interest in activity.

On entry to Woodcroft he was at times able to show and respond to expressions of affection through physical contact, and to appear cheerful and even smile occasionally. On medical records he was summarized as registered blind, with global developmental delay and no useful vision.

His new parents' concerns for him, and their assessment of his special educational needs, were set out in a statutory education department assessment questionnaire as follows:

Q. What worries you most about your child?
Tom's emotional problems concern us most, as they affect his ability to develop in all other areas. He has unpredictable periods of angry, violent behaviour, and although he has begun to make relationships with some adults, he still finds this very difficult, and prefers to be alone for long periods. He prefers not to use language, although he has the ability to use it in a limited manner.

Q. What do you think your child's special education needs are?
1. He is extremely emotionally damaged, and exhibits many signs of autism, including extremely violent, difficult behaviour.
2. His development is very delayed.
3. He is totally blind.
4. He is an adopted child.

Tom's size and general appearance seemed within normal limits for his age; however, it was almost immediately discernible that he had cataracts in both eyes and was constantly moving restlessly and babbling and chattering, chiefly unintelligibly but with the occasional clear, though rarely contextual, word or short phrase, *e.g.* 'no dinner', 'go in car'. He moved about reasonably confidently, testing his surroundings with his hands and feet. He made idiosyncratic verbal connections with what was being said, or with what he understood to be going on, picking up and sometimes repeating key words and phrases, and seemingly jumping to conclusions about the likely nature of his surroundings and destinations. He would appear to estimate his situation verbally in his own jargon and then confirm by tapping and touching with his feet, arms and legs, sometimes rejecting and sometimes eagerly seeking what was on offer. He was subject to outbursts of negative emotional behaviour and distressed protests which were often violent. He would flail with his arms and thrash with his legs, head-butt, grasp and clamber up people, biting, scratching and uttering demand sounds and some echolalic phrases in an occasionally tortured, loud voice.

Initial stage: transfer and entry
Tom was placed in the Primary Class teacher's care and in the direct handling of a male teacher's assistant. This individual was selected from available staff as most appropriate because Tom's previous teacher, with whom he had a close relationship, had been a man of similar presence.

The transfer from school to school was very gradual. Our teacher, assistant, head teacher and speech therapist had all visited his previous school to observe him on several occasions, and the speech therapist had visited his home. Tom had visited this school, initially with his first teacher, and then with a care assistant with whom he had also developed a close relationship. These former staff worked alongside Tom for four or five visits, and then left him in our care. He attended full time. For the first year his original head teacher acted as support teacher twice a week.

Initially, the customary procedure of restricting a child's area to a classroom and its immediate offices was followed (see above). These early days for Tom were summer days, and the garden appealed to him and proved to be an important resource in giving him confidence to move about freely. With careful guidance he learnt his way about, by the slope of the land, the position of trees and shrubs, and the feel of grass, paving stones and gravel. Within days he was steadily leading another blind child by the hand to explore the garden. In the same way, inside the building he soon familiarized himself with the layout of the classroom and its supporting rooms under the guidance of his assistant.

Meals, music sessions and classroom activities soon became a lure into and around other parts of the school building and garden. Another room leading to the garden from the classroom was the first to be made available to Tom to be explored and included in his territory. Eventually, over not more than a month, he was able to be introduced to the rest of the school building as he became aware of succeeding rooms, by hearing intriguing sounds from them, or as he was taken off to the physiotherapy or computer rooms, his assistant always in attendance.

Introductions to the therapists and technicians were also made gradually, but reasonably swiftly, as Tom proved quite eager to relate to new people, as long as he could test the presence of his assistant close at hand by touch and vocal response. He was 'talked through' his school day, and his own vocal responses were listened and responded to.

Formulation of the programme
Detailed reports on the observations summarized above were discussed at the first planning

meeting, held six weeks after admission, with the parents, paediatrician, educational psychologist, representatives from the social services care centre, previous head teacher, the psychotherapist at the clinic and school staff. Tom's strengths and needs as assessed at this stage were presented on the occupational therapist's lists:

Strengths
– Is able to adapt quite quickly to new people, tasks and situations.
– Enjoys physical contact; will seek an adult or peer and initiate interaction.
– Has good gross motor skills generally, although hampered by his visual impairment.
– Will familiarize himself with his surroundings and is able to remember small details of room layouts.
– Locates source and nature of a wide variety of sound.
– Explores objects with all senses available to him.
– Has good manipulative skills, although not always directed or purposeful.
– His vocabulary, although confined to familiar words and phrases, is quite varied, and sentences picked up in an 'echolalic manner' are used appropriately at times.
– Is able to form relationships with people; will react appropriately, and will ask for a specific person or activity.
– Enjoys some puzzles and games, *e.g.* shape sorters, pop-up farm.

Needs
– To develop tactile and fine finger coordination in an appropriate and functional direction (*e.g.* pre-braille work).
– Opportunities to explore and use a range of gross motor skills appropriately, *e.g.* climbing, sliding, go-karting, etc.
– Encouragement to continue to initiate verbalization and to build on his responses.
– Encouragement to be more independent, especially in dressing and eating.
– Opportunities to make choices.
– To extend interest in play equipment and activities, and reduce dependence on certain items.
– Encouragement to participate, take turns, wait and listen during group activities.
– Time to familiarize himself on entering rooms/situations.
– Opportunities to utilize his sense of humour and fun.

Goals
– To bring the concept of sequence into all relevant activities.
– To encourage the formation of concepts and reinforce associated language.
– To provide opportunities for stimulation of all senses (with pre-braille work in mind).
– To motivate him to take initiatives.
– To increase his independence skills.

Adult tasks
– To facilitate the above goals.
– To provide opportunities for exploration and multisensory stimulation.
– To observe and note responses on a continual assessment basis.
– To ensure tasks and activities include an element of enjoyment to encourage motivation.
– To make everything offered meaningful to him.

A curriculum was drawn up, no area being thought inappropriate on the full general curriculum described above, and this has been able to be followed and expanded to provide a reasonably balanced and effective programme.

Delivery of the programme

The delivery of Tom's programme was carefully structured step by step and on a one-to-one, or sometimes two staff to one, basis. For example, if we wanted to encourage sound–hand–eye coordination through rolling a sounding ball, his teacher and his assistant would need to work together with him: one to roll the ball and one to take him through receiving it. If we wanted to reduce his agitated and obsessive rocking, combined with fierce head banging, his teacher would sit with him seated between her legs with his back against her, and join in his rocking until she could sense her way into a slower, less agitated rhythm and perhaps move on to relaxation, a cuddle and finally a happily shared activity, such as walking hand in hand, and so on to a new activity chosen together.

Constant physical reassurance was given, from offering a hand to hold, to stroking his head, hugging and cuddling him; and he was addressed in a voice with calm, friendly tones. During his tantrums he was given space, held if possible in a comforting way to make him feel safe, and then gradually spoken to and introduced to an activity as described above.

Tom's reported 'fits' had to be taken into consideration, and on those school-days when one had taken place at home or on the journey to school, care was taken to follow his pace and be ready to offer the time he needed to recover his equilibrium and reestablish his confidence. He never experienced a seizure in school.

The method of presentation of the programme for Tom at first closely involved his teacher or assistant in therapy sessions, and a timetable had to be gradually devised which was constant and balanced to allow for his concentration span and the need to follow his lead into activity. The detailed components of everything on offer were chosen to have meaning for him and relevance to his experience and needs.

Alongside any observable improvement, Tom continued to exhibit new behaviours which interfered with his progress and which had to be addressed as they occurred. For instance, obsessions and phases came and went; he dominated the scene vocally, shouting phrases at the top of his voice; he interrupted adults' plans for him, for instance by inappropriately and constantly dabbling in and drinking the water during his hand washing programme. As a result, adaptations had to be made to his programme, and in some cases to the environment, in order to try to find a positive way forward.

In our experience, it is at home that children learn most, and in Tom's case the vital ability to trust has been fostered, and the expression of his feelings awakened and encouraged, by his adoptive parents' devotion to him and to his welfare and many and varied needs. Many of his advances in life skills have been initiated at home, and detailed comments and reports of activities have been passed between home and school via his daily diary and at regular visits to school by his mother and father.

Outcome

The outcome of our proffered educational and therapeutic interventions is difficult to evaluate, but for a period in Tom's life we tried to share some of the demands imposed upon him and his parents by his blindness and other disabilities. For all concerned—including the paediatrician who visited him regularly and remained constantly involved, and the psycho-therapist whom he continued to see regularly—trying to maintain an awareness of his needs and to reach a consensus about how best to address those needs was an essential part of the programme.

Despite all his problems, Tom developed a sense of humour and found many reasons to laugh and express joy. His ability to trust people and to give affection, previously limited mainly to his parents, grew to encompass others outside the home, including workers at the clinic, the support team of social workers and many of the staff in school.

Conclusion

A programme for the multiply disabled, visually impaired child should meet that child's needs through the offer of appropriate teaching and therapy. If it is to be effective, an atmosphere of trust between the school and the child and her/his family is vital, and no effort should be spared in trying to develop that trust. The programme must remain flexible, and should be sensitive to the need of the child to be respected and valued for her/his own sake. In addition, parents' hopes, fears, wishes and expertise need to be acknowledged, and their involvement fostered and appreciated throughout.

We have found that such a programme needs to be constantly monitored and evaluated for appropriateness and effectiveness. It should take into account that a child with severe visual impairment cannot learn by visual patterning on her/his peers, and that appropriate intervention at a point of readiness is essential, often on a one-to-one basis and for as long as is necessary.

In order to benefit from the programme, the child must be interested, and suitably relaxed and confident that her/his efforts will be accepted. In addition, s/he should be encouraged to have sufficient self-esteem and satisfaction in achievement to continue to be willing to cooperate with the efforts being made on her/his behalf.

Members of the teaching and therapy team also need a similar sense of their own value to the child and to one another, and a relaxed and supportive environment within which to function. They need to know their strengths and should consult on a daily basis and be constantly ready to change approaches in order to formulate the strategies most likely to prove effective in achieving for the child the optimum level of maturity.

REFERENCE

Gunzburg, H.C. (1973) *Progress Assessment Chart*. Stratford-upon-Avon: SEFA.

BIBLIOGRAPHY

Aitken, S., Buultjens, M. (1992) *Vision for Doing: Assessing Functional Vision of Learners Who Are Multiply Disabled*. Edinburgh: Moray House.
Book, W.F. (1908) *The Psychology of Skill*. (Reprinted 1973, New York: Arno Press.)
Freud, A. (1965) *Normality and Pathology in Childhood*. New York: International Universities Press.
Garvey, C. (1977) *Play*. Cambridge, MA: Harvard University Press.
Gesell, A. (1954) *The First Five Years of Life*. London: Methuen.
Isaacs, S. (1933) *Social Development in Young Children*. London: Routledge.
Kellmer Pringle, M. (1974) *The Needs of Children*. London: Hutchinson.
Liedloff, J. (1986) *The Continuum Concept. Revised Edn.* Harmondsworth: Penguin.
Lovaas, I. (1981) *Teaching Developmentally Disabled Children*. Tunbridge Wells, Kent: Costello Educational.
McKendrick, O. (1991) *Assessment of Multi-handicapped Visually Impaired Children*. London: RNIB.
Myklebust, H.R. (1964) *The Psychology of Deafness, Sensory Deprivation, Learning and Adjustment*. London: Grune & Stratton.
Nielsen, L. (1990) *Are You Blind? Promotion of the Development of Children Who Are Especially Developmentally Threatened*. Copenhagen: Sikon.

Piaget, J. (1959) *The Language and Thought of the Child. Children's Developmental Progress.* London: Routledge & Kegan Paul.

Rutter, M. (1991) *Maternal Deprivation Reassessed.* Harmondsworth: Penguin.

Sebba, J. (1980) *A System for Assessment and Intervention for Pre-school Profoundly Retarded Multiply Handicapped Children.* Manchester: Hester Adrian Research Centre.

Sheridan, M. (1973) *From Birth to Five Years. The Stycar Sequences.* Windsor: NFER.

Simon, G.B. (1973) *The Next Step on the Ladder.* Kidderminster: British Institute of Mental Handicap.

Valentine, C.W. (1913) *An Introduction to Experimental Psychology.* London: University Tutorial Press.

Vygotsky, L.S. (1933) 'Play and its role in the mental development of the child.' (*Reprinted 1976 in:* Bruner, J., Jolly, A., Sylva, K. (Eds) *Play: Its Role in Development and Evolution.* Harmondsworth: Penguin, pp. 58–62.)

Warnock Report (1978) *Special Educational Needs. Report of the Committee of Enquiry into the Education of Handicapped Children and Adults. Command 7212.* London: HMSO.

Winnicott, D.W. (1971) *Playing and Reality.* London: Tavistock.

—— (1971/1985) *Creativity and its Origins.* New York: Basic Books; Harmondsworth: Penguin.

11
THE EDUCATIONAL IMPLICATIONS OF VISUAL IMPAIRMENT

Michael J. Tobin

This chapter draws attention to some of the effects that severe visual impairment can have on the educational progress of blind and partially sighted children. As revealed by the RNIB survey (Walker *et al.* 1992), there are also differences in the ways in which families react to the birth of a child with an impairment of sight, and these reactions can themselves have direct and indirect implications for the child's education. An attempt to summarize even the direct educational effects is fraught with difficulties, due in the main to the heterogeneity of the causations, symptoms and sequelae. For example, some albino children will have few difficulties in the normal classroom environment but may experience great discomfort in bright outdoor situations for physical education classes or when indoors for drama and movement lessons in conditions of high illumination. For other children, reduced visual fields may be associated with relatively good distant or near acuities, allowing satisfactory progress in the development of reading accuracy skills, while also being associated with much below-average reading speeds. Total blindness will of course have educational implications of an altogether different kind, involving radically different teaching approaches and radically different learning methods.

The World Health Organization's recommended definitions of impairment, disability and handicap (Table 11.1) are useful in forcing us to ask the right questions about the educational implications of blindness and severe visual impairment since they point to the importance of the specific social, educational and vocational 'contexts' for assessing whether or not a particular impairment is likely to have handicapping consequences. In many learning situations the impairment will not be predicted to have such consequences, while in others even a quite minor degree of impairment will be severely disabling and will result in a significant handicap. For example, the child with myopia will be handicapped when deciphering words and diagrams on the blackboard but not when reading 12- or even 10-point print in a well-designed textbook. Nevertheless, before identifying some of the specific handicaps stemming from specific impairments in specific contexts, it may be useful to examine the extent to which any degree of visual disability might interfere with a child's understanding of the objects and phenomena of her/his physical and social worlds.

Teachers of blind and partially sighted children often stumble across gaps in the general knowledge and experience of these children, gaps which they attribute

TABLE 11.1

WHO definitions of impairments, disabilities and handicaps*

Impairment: any loss or abnormality of psychological, physiological or anatomical structure or function.

Disability: any restriction or lack (resulting from an impairment) of ability to perform an activity in the manner or within the range considered normal for a human being.

Handicap: a disadvantage for a given individual, resulting from an impairment or disability, that limits or prevents the fulfilment of a role (depending on age, sex, and social and cultural factors) for that individual.

*World Health Organization (1980)

to the children's failure to perceive similarities, differences and invariances. For the fully sighted child, the everyday world presents quite gratuitously numerous examples of objects that are perceptually different in terms of colour, shape and size but which are nevertheless functionally 'the same'. The following anecdotes illustrate these kinds of gaps in learning:

John was six years old, totally blind from birth. He and his teacher were walking, hand in hand, through the garden of the school. As they neared a silver birch tree his teacher said: 'Let's feel this tree, this plant'. She placed both his hands on the trunk of the tree. He moved them over the bark and then slid them right round the trunk until they met and his face was touching the bark: 'Coo, what a big pot it must be growing in!'

Mary was 14 years old, with very little residual vision and with some other moderate physical and learning disabilities. In the process of preparing for the school's Christmas party, her teacher asked her to place some loaves of bread on the tables. On returning to the refectory, the teacher saw Mary standing in the same place, doing nothing: 'Oh, Mary, do be of some use. Put the loaves out'. In the time honoured way, the teacher went away, came back yet again, saw that Mary had not moved from the spot, and said: 'Mary, for goodness sake, do try to be helpful. Put the loaves on the tables'. 'But, Miss, you haven't given me the bread. Where are the loaves?' Mary was already holding four unwrapped, well-baked, crusty loaves, but for her, loaves were pre-sliced objects, wrapped in grease-proof paper. (Tobin 1992, p. 178)

For John, a plant was an object with which he was very familiar: it grew in a pot. Unfortunately his blindness had thus far debarred him from perceiving a 'family of likenesses' among the myriad kinds of plants, such that enable us to classify them all as plants. Similarly, Mary had no experience of handling a traditional loaf of bread. Both children were bound by the particular features that had greatest sensory salience for them. With fully-sighted children, teachers and parents work on the assumption that they will generalize the concept, and its verbal label, to the many other, often perceptually dissimilar, exemplars of that concept. They do not expect to have to draw the child's attention to every chair or table or plant, and teach her/him that this also is a chair, a table, a plant. It is not possible for teachers to draw up an exhaustive checklist that can be used to explore the gaps in a child's experiences, but it will be recognized that such gaps can interfere with the

144

acquisition and formation of some of the prerequisite concepts and operations of elementary mathematics and science, and indeed of most of the conventional areas of the school curriculum.

Seriation in mathematics illustrates the point nicely. Most young sighted children will have built towers of wooden or plastic blocks, learning, usually without any formal teaching, that a stable tower can only be built if the largest block is at the bottom, with the others being piled up in descending order of size. Such casual, unplanned behaviour—complemented by apparently passive observation of other people engaged upon similar activities—will often be beyond the blind child's experience. Countless repetitions of these kinds of activities form the concrete basis for the notion of ordering, of seriation. The blind child's acquisition and then complete mastery of the underlying concepts and operations cannot be taken for granted merely because s/he demonstrates understanding in a particular situation and can use the appropriate words. It needs an experienced and alert teacher to probe what lies behind the surface familiarity.

Other gaps in experience may arise from the characteristics of the communication medium used by the blind learner. The highly condensed nature of Standard English Braille results in many words and letter groupings being expressed by a single tactile symbol. For example, when the braille sign for the letter K is written with a space in front and after it, it represents the word 'knowledge'. In the ordinary course of reading and writing, the braillist will not be forced to remember how to spell knowledge, nor, indeed, a host of other words (such as 'character', 'ought', 'their' and 'there') that are often misspelled by fully sighted print-readers. The absence of daily exposure by the braillist to the many orthographical irregularities of English can lead to poor spelling when the blind student is required to learn typewriting for communicating with sighted teachers, friends and relatives.

As shown in Figure 11.1, braille places other perceptual and cognitive demands on the learner: the same tactile sign can have different meanings, the determining factor being the sign's position on the line or in the string of letters.

The valuable space-saving qualities of fully contracted braille can therefore have an educational and vocational impact. Its resolution has implications for teaching, involving extra time and effort being expended by teachers and learners, possibly at the expense of achieving other important educational objectives.

Among the skills acquired in the course of education is the ability to represent the three-dimensional physical world by means of two-dimensional drawings—maps, diagrams, graphs. Data are compressed and condensed so that the information is conveyed in its totality. Vision then allows the whole 'scene' to be grasped virtually immediately, and makes possible rapid and repeated comparisons among the discrete elements of the array. When such diagrams are in a tactile form, their deciphering requires a sequential scanning, with successive pieces of information having to be held in 'temporary store' until enough has been registered to permit complete identification. Apart from the demands made on short-term memory capacity—a capacity that grows steadily throughout childhood—there is

(i) The basic braille cell consists of 6 dots:

●●
●●
●●

(ii) The sign

○○
●●
○●   stands for:

dis at the beginning of a string of letters
dd in the middle of a string of letters
Full stop at the end of a string of letters.

(iii) The same shape, but higher up in the cell

●●
○●
○○   stands for:

d at the beginning, in the middle, and at the end of a string of letters.
do when spaced from all other signs.

Fig. 11.1. Standard English Braille: meaning determined by position.

also the problem of maintaining a frame of reference. For the sighted child, the external coordinates of x and y axes, tops and bottoms of pages, and the cardinal points of the compass, all serve to provide stable frames of reference. This easy comparison with fixed parameters is not so readily available to the blind child. Merely maintaining a straight left-to-right or up and down scanning of the page is problematical, making the comparison of the heights of adjacent bar graphs or the points in a frequency polygon extremely difficult. The heavy demands upon short-term memory and psychomotor skills can be compounded by the sometimes poor quality of the tactile signs: insufficient differences in the height, width and shape of the embossments make recognition either impossible or inordinately long drawn out.

Although there are now well-proven methods for producing high quality embossed materials (see, for example, Hinton 1988), there is a need for blind children to be given training in the systematic scanning and exploration of tactile diagrams. This, in turn, has to be superimposed upon early tactile exploration of three-dimensional objects, with parents and teachers using their own and the child's developing language skills for drawing attention to such notions as

146

TABLE 11.2

Mean oral reading speed ages* of two groups of partially sighted learners

	Mean chrono-logical age (yrs:mths)	Mean reading speed age (yrs:mths)	Mean deficit (yrs:mths)
Group 1 (N = 43)	9:4	8:2	1:2
Group 2 (N = 51)	11:10	8:10	3:0

*As assessed using the Neale Analysis of Reading Ability (Neale 1966).

roundness, straightness and discontinuity; to such significant features as vertices and edges; and to the ways in which there are similarities and differences when these features are represented in the quasi-two dimensionality of tactile drawings. Instruction in these matters is part of the visually disabled learner's additional curriculum. Failure to recognize that such provision has to be made will act as a brake upon the blind child's progress; formal recognition of its importance entails additional time slots being built into an already over-burdened syllabus. This 'no win' situation brings out quite starkly some of the educationally handicapping consequences of blindness.

Additional curricular requirements constitute a considerable burden for parents, teachers and learners. Many of them can be seen as prerequisites for competence in the traditional subjects and activities of the curriculum, but there are others, such as long-cane mobility training, typewriting, self-care, and social and daily living skills, that do not directly impinge on the learning of science, mathematics and geography but that are essential if the child is to be able to function independently as a member of the school. They take up time, and the danger is that, in making space for them, other subjects are either dropped or studied to a lower level than is within the learner's compass. It is not so much a case of the visual impairment directly interfering with the child's learning, as of the educational logistics of matching the learner's needs and ambitions with the time and teaching skills that are available.

If gaps in experience and the problems of organizing additional teaching are potential causes of educational handicap for the blind child, is the position the same for the child who is not blind but whose vision is so poor that s/he is registrable as partially sighted? For many such children, residual vision may be good enough for them to cope with ink-print, to dispense with formal mobility training, and to be able to learn social and daily living skills by imitation, that is by copying the actions and behaviour of their sighted parents, teachers and age-peers. For these visually impaired learners, the major educational problem is likely to be the much slower rate of information processing. This will manifest itself most clearly in speed of reading. Table 11.2 reports data from an ongoing study (by the present author) of the reading skills of children registered as partially sighted and attending special schools for the visually impaired. Mean oral reading speeds in two different age-groups are compared with the normative data for fully sighted readers. These show clearly the effects of their visual impairments on their ability to process visually presented materials. At a mean chronological age of 9 years 4 months, the pupils in the first group were on average 14 months behind their sighted peers; at a mean chronological age of 11 years 10 months, the second group's deficit was of the order of 36 months.

Deficits of these orders of magnitude point to a specific educational disadvantage experienced by these visually impaired children. Not only will they take longer than their fully sighted peers to work their way through set texts in literature, they will also be disadvantaged when tackling tasks in, for instance, geography, history or science which involve scanning back and forth to locate instructions and key words and phrases. While spectacles, contact lenses, closed circuit TV magnifiers, and other low vision aids will help to make text and diagrams clearer for them, those children who have to operate very close to the text will often continue to be decoding such materials at much slower speeds than their classmates.

Different samples of partially sighted readers will undoubtedly show differing levels of competence, but current studies by the present author are revealing the same overall pattern of deficit in terms of the speed of processing of visually presented materials. For the blind child who is dependent upon braille, the picture is similar: a massive disadvantage in speed, and one that seems to become greater throughout early adolescence just at the time when the learner is being expected to become less dependent upon her/his teachers and when the quantity of reading is growing rapidly.

Despite the educational handicaps that may be caused directly by severe visual impairment or that can arise indirectly from the characteristics of the special communication methods (braille and large print) or that also stem indirectly from the need to learn additional skills, the education of blind and partially sighted learners is full of exciting possibilities. Modern technology can do much to mitigate the difficulties. Computer-controlled visual display units can optimize the visual environment by allowing learners to alter the size of print on the screen, to choose levels of brightness and contrast, and to select preferred colours of background and foreground images (see, for example, Hawley *et al.* 1987, Spencer and Ross 1989, Bozic 1992, Bozic *et al.* 1993). Totally blind students can use specially designed software that enables them to braille or type assignments, with printed output for their teachers and braille copies for their own files, while editing and corrections can be done without recourse to sighted helpers now that access to what is printed on the screen can be effected by means of synthetic speech (Campbell and Vallender 1992). This new technology is discussed further in Chapter 14.

Information technology is not in itself sufficient to eradicate the educationally handicapping consequences of visual impairment. Specific skills teaching—for improving reading speeds, for example—requires that teachers are both know-

148

ledgeable about the skills and experienced in teaching the learners. It is the teacher who can observe and assess the particular need, whether it be for a variable speed tape recorder to facilitate the revision of lengthy texts, for additional time allowances in public examinations, or for activities that will make good the gaps in basic knowledge and learning.

Fortunately, there has been an increase in the numbers of specialist teachers (see Chapman and Stone 1988), and this is now making it possible for more and more visually impaired children to be integrated and taught in neighbourhood, mainstream schools or within specialist units attached to such schools. This development widens, at least in principle, the range of choices available to families. The goal of meeting individual and differentiated needs is what is aimed at by all those involved in the education of children suffering from severe defects of vision, and the availability of specially qualified and experienced teachers is the prerequisite for its attainment.

REFERENCES

Bozic, N. (1992) 'Using joystick software with visually impaired children: Part 2.' *Eye Contact*, **4**, 17–19.
—— Hill, E.W., Tobin, M.J. (1993) 'Pre-school visually impaired children: visual stimulation and micro-computers.' *Child: Care, Health and Development*, **19**, 25–35.
Campbell, S.L., Vallender, M.D. (1992) 'Modern technology: access to print for blind and partially sighted people.' *Computer Education*, **71**, 6–8.
Chapman, E.K., Stone, J.M. (1988) *The Visually Handicapped Child in Your Classroom*. London: Cassell.
Hawley, A., Jefferys, S., Ross, M., Spencer, S., Tobin, M.J. (1987) 'Electronic publishing and visually handicapped learners.' *The New Beacon*, LXXI, 844, 253–255.
Hinton, R. (1988) *New Ways with Diagrams: Thermoformed Tactile Diagrams—a Manual for Teachers and Technicians*. London: RNIB.
Neale, M.D. (1966) *Neale Analysis of Reading Ability: Manual of Directions and Norms. 2nd Edn*. London: Macmillan.
Spencer, S., Ross, M. (1989) 'Software packages for the young visually handicapped.' *Special Children*, **31**, 20–21.
Tobin, M.J. (1992) 'The language of blind children: communication, words, and meanings.' *Language and Education*, **6**, 177–182.
Walker, E., Tobin, M.J., McKennell, A. (1992) *Blind and Partially Sighted Children in Britain: the RNIB Survey*. London: HMSO.
World Health Organization (1980) *International Classification of Impairments, Disabilities and Handicaps. A Manual of Classification*. Geneva: WHO.

12
EDUCATING THE MULTIPLY DISABLED BLIND CHILD

Judy Bell

Introduction

The education of the multiply disabled blind child provides the educator with a particular set of challenges. Before addressing these challenges it is important to clarify two issues:

• *What is meant by blindness in this context?*

In a population where precision in the testing of vision is problematic, definitions of the categories of visual impairment are difficult. Within an educational context classification according to measurement is probably less useful than definitions involving a descriptive element. Therefore, the term 'blind' is taken here to refer to those children who do not use their sight for any purpose but rely wholly on alternative means of sensory input. It includes children who have serious occular malformations or damage, those with a neurological basis for their impairment and those who are not using their available sight.

• *What is meant by multiple disability?*

As Chapman and Stone (1988) point out, current educational thinking has moved away from the idea of labelling children according to categories of 'handicap'. Each child has a unique pattern of abilities, skills, impairments and disabilities which will give rise to a personal set of educational needs. These needs will be dependent not only on the severity and types of impairment but also on the child's age and maturity at the time of onset, motivation, personality, self-concept, life experiences, and the quality and relevance of the educational opportunities which have been available.

From an educational standpoint, therefore, multiply disabled blind children do not form a single, homogeneous group. A small number of such children will be functioning at an age-appropriate level and will be able to benefit from modified means of access to a full mainstream curriculum. A much larger number of children will be operating at a level which is developmentally severely delayed. Some of the issues arising from the meeting of the educational needs of these latter children are addressed in this chapter.

The effect of blindness on educational need

It is generally recognized that vision is the major coordinating sense (Zinkin 1979), so that where it is absent the child will have a seriously decreased ability to integrate into a meaningful whole the information which is received through the other senses. If this information is itself incomplete or distorted as a result of other impairments, or if the ability to integrate it is flawed, then the child's needs will be complex. S/he will have real difficulties in achieving a balanced understanding of the environment and of her/his position within it. It is the task of the educator to manipulate the variables which are available within an educational context to maximize the opportunities for the development of this understanding.

One can consider the following variables as the means by which the educator can bring about an effective means of meeting the educational needs of multiply disabled blind children:

- the environment in which education is provided;
- the forms of assessment used;
- the teaching approach(es) adopted;
- the content of, and access to, the curriculum;
- the channels of communication between parents and professionals.

Educational environment

The educational environment for multiply disabled blind children will need especial attention. The absence of the integrating sense of vision will mean that it is particularly hard for such children to discriminate those aspects of their surroundings which are meaningful and those which are not. The organization of both the temporal and spatial environments must allow for the maximum derivation of meaning and understanding. In addition, the opportunities for incidental learning will be reduced by the lack of sight (Best 1986), and there is a need to organize the environment to ensure that such incidental learning as does occur is orderly and significant. A discussion of some of the practical issues involved is provided by Bethell and Bell (1984). Factors which require consideration include: levels of auditory, tactile and olfactory distraction; routines of activities having a regular occurrence; timetabling and sequencing of activities; spatial arrangements of people and objects; and the type, qualities and position of furniture.

Forms of assessment

For many years there has been an awareness among educators that skill-based assessments provide a valuable means both of recording achievements and of planning what to do (or not to do) next. Best (1987) identifies four main purposes of assessment for teachers of young visually impaired children; these are equally applicable to those concerned with the education of the multiply disabled blind child: (1) the establishment of a baseline for teaching; (2) the recording of changes in performance over time; (3) the identification of teaching steps; (4) the provision of ideas for learning activities.

If maximum benefit is to derive to the child it is imperative that the form of the assessment used is appropriate to the circumstances of the child and to the purposes for which it is required by the educator. Information deriving from assessment is unlikely to be useful in either guiding teaching or recording progress if the incremental steps between skills are so large as to be inappropriate for a child with a slow rate of skill acquisition. Similarly, assessment will be of little practical use in the school if it is based purely on the acquisition of skills by a fully sighted, fully ambulant child, with no flexibility of recording to allow for unique combinations of impairments. If the teacher were to stick rigidly to such a procedure it is likely that the learning experiences offered to the child would be inappropriate to her/his needs. Best and Bell (1984) provide an analysis of 12 schedules used to assess children who are profoundly disabled, and Best (1988) reviews procedures used with young visually impaired children, some of which will also be appropriate to the multiply disabled blind child.

There can be no single prescription of assessment procedures. To be useful, it seems clear that they must be relevant to the population and to the circumstances. It is not the choice of procedures alone which affects the education that is offered. The manner of translation from assessed skills to learning experiences will both affect, and be affected by, the teaching approaches that are employed.

Teaching approaches

In many countries an important impact has been, and continues to be, made by the application of behavioural approaches to the teaching of multiply disabled children, including those who are blind. Best (1986) notes that the presence of a visual impairment affects decisions but not the processes involved in such an approach. The use of a technique which emphasizes clarity of intention through the specification of precise behavioural objectives and criteria of performance together with the breaking down of skills into small component steps has been widely held to be of significant value in teaching new skills to those whose ability to acquire such skills incidentally is severely impeded. The nature of what is taught may be affected by the individual's visual impairment but the techniques remain valid. This behavioural approach to teaching is highly dependent on the use of skills checklists which are used in the selection and specification of tasks. These checklists may already be broken down so that each step represents a small learning task, although for some children there may need to be a further analysis of the steps involved in the acquisition of a given skill.

While it is recognized that the behavioural approach has much to offer, Sebba and Hogg (1988) note that there is a growing recognition of a need to extend teaching beyond the rigid application of behavioural principles. Bray *et al.* (1988) provide an eloquent argument for a more interactive, less teacher-controlled approach, in which increased value is placed on the initiations of the child. The emphasis here is on the processes and nature of the learning experiences themselves rather than on predetermined outcomes of child behaviour as prescribed by a checklist. In this context assessment will still be useful but the emphasis will be more on the establishment of a baseline for teaching and in the recording of changes in performance over time.

This interactive approach is embodied in the teaching within a number of schools, notably at the Royal National Institute for the Blind's School for children with visual and other disabilities at Rushton Hall, Northamptonshire, UK, as described by Sharron (1987). At this school the staff have eschewed conventional objectives-led ـbehavioural teaching for an approach which recognizes the importance of 'bonding' between adult and child. There is an emphasis on teaching in context rather than in what can be considered as artificially created situations in the classroom (Wood 1990). This raises the issue of the place of education. With this more interactive, naturalistic approach, teaching must be viewed as continuing at all times in all places. It is not an activity which is the sole prerogative of the teacher in the classroom. The role of parents and care-givers cannot, therefore, be considered as divorced from that of the educator.

In view of the vast range of skills and behaviours which the educator is required to address, a pluralistic approach drawing on both behavioural and interactive philosophy would seem to be appropriate. Where skills require a high level of mechanical practice for their emergence and refinement, such as in the area of self-help, behavioural techniques seem particularly useful. Where skills depend for their development on interactive processes, such as in the area of language, an approach with an emphasis on facilitation rather than prescription might be appropriate. However, it is unlikely that universal agreement over relative methods will ever be reached, and the proponents of each will have strongly held views regarding their applicability to the education of the multiply disabled blind child.

Content of, and access to, the curriculum
In England and Wales, the 1988 Education Reform Act introduced a 'national curriculum' for all pupils between the ages of 5 and 16 years. This has raised many interesting and far-reaching questions in relation to its applicability to the education of children with special needs, in particular those with multiple disabilities who are operating at a delayed developmental level. Although the requirements of the curriculum can be set aside or modified through a formal procedure, there is a widespread feeling that to do so would delineate a population which is incapable of benefiting from education. This would mark a return to the situation which prevailed in England and Wales prior to the 1970 Education (Handicapped Children) Act. Before the passing of this Act some children were classified as suffering from such a 'disability of mind' as to make them unsuitable for education in any local education authority school. Such children were considered 'ineducable', and their care, treatment and training were held to be the responsibility of health, rather than education authorities. Whatever position is adopted by schools in relation to the demands of the national curriculum, the underpinning principle that the curriculum should be 'broad, balanced and relevant' will have implications for multiply disabled blind children. In the past the educational needs of such children have sometimes been interpreted as requiring a content heavily weighted to practical elements concerned with the basics of self-

care, such as feeding, dressing and toileting, to assist in a future of planned dependence. While such content is relevant, it is neither broad nor balanced. Nevertheless, if individual needs are to be met by education it is important that such skills are still addressed by schools' curricula.

The means of access to the curriculum will need to take into account the child's available sensory channels and the levels of development, refinement and sensitivity which have been achieved. Teaching must use a combination of tactile, auditory, gustatory and kinaesthetic inputs in order to provide the child with maximal access to the full curriculum content. In so doing the following points must be born in mind. (1) Some children will have reduced sensation in other sensory channels. (2) The ability to integrate sensations may be impaired. (3) There will have been reduced opportunities to experience and explore the properties of objects. (4) More time will be necessary for acquiring information in the absence of vision.

It is likely that some children will have to be taught how to use their senses in order to access the curriculum. The development and training of such skills will necessitate areas of content which are specific to the needs of multiply disabled blind children.

Two further areas require consideration in relation to multiply disabled blind children: mobility and visual stimulation.

MOBILITY

Those blind children who have difficulties in movement or who are wheelchair dependent are likely to have very specific needs. These will be related to the understanding of space and their own orientation within it. Specific mobility training will be just as vital for them as for those who are able to benefit from more formal long-cane training. If this is not addressed it is likely that the child's understanding of space will extend no further, and possibly not even as far, as the tiny area around their own body. For those children who are capable of independent movement a useful discussion of ideas for mobility training is provided by Harley and Hill (1986). The importance of senses other than vision and hearing to mobility and orientation training are highlighted by Murdoch (1989) in her description of teaching a totally deaf–blind child to move around with confidence.

VISUAL STIMULATION

Although stimulating the vision of a blind person may seem a contradiction in terms, there is a widespread feeling among teachers of multiply disabled children that programmes of visual stimulation have a beneficial effect. Children who have a cortical visual impairment or those who fall into the category described by Jose *et al.* (1980) of being unaware that they have any vision may benefit from the kind of intervention described by Mabon (1988) involving the use of lights, movement and patterns. Many schools now have well equipped dark- or light-rooms which provide the environment for the necessary manipulation of lighting and the isolation of

154

visual stimuli. Without such facilities the implementation of these programmes is difficult. Despite the enthusiasm with which such activities are included in the curricula of schools, there is little empirical evidence of the value of such interventions (Erin 1986).

Channels of communication between parents and professionals
For learning to be generalized, for practical problems of management to be minimized and for a consistency of expectation and handling to be achieved, good communication is necessary between parents and professionals involved in the education of multiply disabled blind children. It is inevitable that there is a blurring of responsibility between home and school. Educators and parents have a shared responsibility for the development of skills which will be applicable in a variety of situations. They may each have to tackle the same kinds of problem behaviours, and they will jointly have to decide on priorities for intervention.

Lambe and Sebba (1988) suggest that the organization of workshops will provide an economical method of transferring information and expertise to families of profoundly disabled children. That such activities will be useful is beyond doubt. However, it should be borne in mind that the transfer of information is not just a one-way process. Parents are likely to know aspects of their child's personality, skills and behaviours that are unobserved by the professionals. A full repertoire of formal and informal communication procedures will be necessary, including home–school diaries, video recordings, telephone calls, workshops, meetings, profiles of achievement, visits and even school reports, to facilitate a coordinated approach to meeting the educational needs of these children.

Conclusion
Educating multiply disabled blind children is a complex issue where there are no straightforward or simple courses of action. In this chapter an attempt has been made to address some of the variables which it is possible to isolate and consider in meeting the needs of this population. The particular approach which is adopted will be dependent on the overall philosophy and aims of the school. The effectiveness with which it is implemented will depend on the hard work and dedication of the educator in partnership with parents and care-givers.

REFERENCES

Best, A.B. (1986) 'Approaches to teaching people with visual and mental handicaps.' *In:* Ellis, D. (Ed.) *Sensory Impairments in Mentally Handicapped People.* London: Croom Helm, pp. 339–357.
—— (1987) 'Assessment procedures for use with young visually handicapped children. Part one.' *British Journal of Visual Impairment*, **5**, 85–88.
—— (1988) 'Assessment procedures for use with young visually handicapped children. Part two.' *British Journal of Visual Impairment*, **6**, 7–10.
—— Bell, J. (1984) 'Assessment of children with profound handicaps. An analysis of 12 schedules.' *Mental Handicap*, **12**, 160–163.
Bethell, D., Bell, J. (1984) 'Approaches to curriculum.' *Information Exchange*, **11**, 3–13.

Bray, A., Macarthur, J., Ballard, K.D. (1988) 'Education for pupils with profound disabilities: issues of policy, curriculum, teaching methods and evaluation.' *European Journal of Special Needs in Education*, **3**, 207–224.

Chapman, E.K., Stone, J.M. (1988) *The Visually Handicapped Child in Your Classroom*. London: Cassell.

Erin, J.N. (1986) 'Teachers of the visually handicapped: how can they best serve children with profound handicaps?' *Education of the Visually Handicapped*, **18**, 15–25.

Harley, R.K., Hill, M.M. (1986) 'Mobility training for visually impaired mentally handicapped persons.' *In:* Ellis, D. (Ed.) *Sensory Impairments in Mentally Handicapped People*. London: Croom Helm, pp. 408–426.

Jose, R.T., Smith, A.J., Shane, K.G. (1980) 'Evaluating and stimulating vision in the multiply impaired.' *Journal of Visual Impairment and Blindness*, **74**, 2–8.

Lambe, L., Sebba, J. (1988) 'The development and evaluation of workshops for parents and carers of people with profound and multiple impairments.' *European Journal of Special Needs in Education*, **3**, 257–266.

Mabon, M. (1988) 'Assessment and management of visual development.' *In:* Sebba, J. (Ed.) *The Education of People with Profound and Multiple Handicaps: Resource Materials for Staff Training*, Manchester: Manchester University Press, pp. 110–121.

Murdoch, H. (1989) 'Steps towards mobility.' *Talking Sense*, **35**, 20–22.

Sebba, J., Hogg, J. (1988) 'Introduction. Profound and multiple impairments: an evolving field.' *European Journal of Special Needs in Education*, **3**, 187–188.

Sharron, H. (1987) 'Catching children the state misses: Rushton Hall.' *Special Children*, **15**, 27–29.

Wood, D. (1990) 'Whose needs first?' *Talking Sense*, **36**, 8–9.

Zinkin, P.M. (1979) 'The effect of visual handicap on early development.' *In:* Smith, V., Keen, J. (Eds) *Visual Handicap in Children. Clinics in Developmental Medicine No. 73*. London: Spastics International Medical Publications, pp. 132–138.

13
ACCESS TO THE CURRICULUM FOR CHILDREN WITH VISUAL IMPAIRMENTS

Anthony B. Best

In the 1960s an American scientist, James Bliss, invented a machine that he hoped would help his blind daughter. He wanted her to attend her local primary school but teachers were suggesting, as was common at that time, that she should be sent to a residential special school fully equipped to meet her special needs. Her lack of access to print materials was identified as a major barrier to learning. If she could not read the material that the other children had, this would prevent her placement in the local school. The machine, which Bliss called the Optacon, consists of a hand-held scanner which, when moved over a page of print, converts the shape of each letter into a raised form which can be felt by the fingers of the reader's other hand. In this way a blind child can have direct access to print and thereby read the same materials as other children in the class.

It seemed to be the solution. But, although the machine is still produced today, it was of very little help. The problem of educating a blind child is only partially one of access to print. Much primary school work is based on drawings, pictures, graphs, large posters, demonstrations, video tapes and experiments, none of which can be accessed through the Optacon.

But more fundamentally, the problem is one of access to educational experiences. The child may be able to read words such as wave, pyramid, horizon, chimney, bee and snowflake, but without extra help cannot understand what those words mean. A blind child understands very little of what a wave is—how it forms, moves, breaks—just by reading the word or even listening to the sound of a wave; a common object like a chimney will not be really understood unless the object is directly experienced through touch; the concept of the horizon can only be comprehended through the use of models and careful description. This might compare the visual horizon to experiences with sounds fading in the distance but would emphasize the linear nature of vision compared to the ability of sounds to be heard 'round corners'. Providing such educational experiences is thus a major part of the challenge of educating children with visual impairments.

Take, for example a maths lesson. Children spend very little time simply going through pages of sums. If that were the case, then education would not be so difficult for blind children. They are more likely to be set a problem such as this one. A picture shows a hanging basket of plants supported on a chain by a bracket fastened to a wall, and a bigger and heavier basket which is supported by a longer bracket. The child is asked to work out the design of a support for an even bigger basket. The maths problem is one of ratios and progressions, but for a blind child there are additional difficulties; simply stating the problem in words presents a different task to the child. The blind child is unable to visualize the relationships; there may be other elements in the pictures (*e.g.* the length of the chain) which the sighted child has to eliminate as part of solving the problem; the lack of experience in seeing weights supported by brackets may hinder the blind child's understanding of the situation; having to remember the spoken information is more difficult than being able to study all the examples in one glance.

A visual impairment limits the quality and quantity of a child's experiences and so effects that child's understanding and development. Education must provide access to an appropriate curriculum which will overcome these privations.

There are two elements to the solution. One is the provision of appropriate support to access the regular school curriculum. The second is access to a special curriculum which develops skills, such as mobility and braille, that are needed by the child.

This is the situation whatever type of school the child attends. Today, placement in a local school for sighted children is the preferred option of many parents. For this to be effective, class teachers need support from specially trained visiting teachers who provide advice, some direct teaching and modified learning materials.

The regular curriculum

Children need to have access to the content of the lessons and this requires adaptations to teaching materials, special teaching approaches and the provision of special teachers to identify and overcome the difficulties children may have in understanding the content of the lessons.

Reading and writing is the central difficulty. The majority of children classed as visually impaired are able to use print. Where regular sized print cannot be seen, one method of access is through a low vision aid. These devices usually use one or more lenses to form an optical microscopic or telescopic system which magnifies the image of an object such as a print letter. This allows access to much of the regular material and provides a portable and relatively inexpensive solution. Enlarging photocopiers are also popular as a way of accessing print but this may be because of their convenience in use as they do restrict the child to material that has been specially prepared. The result may be bulky and of inappropriate size print when letters of different sizes are all enlarged to a uniform degree. The enlargement of many diagrams creates images which are too large to be useful.

There are two problems with the preferred method of low vision devices. One is that a significant number of children are reluctant to use the aid in class through a feeling that it will draw attention to them. However unreasonable or petty this may seem, it is a significant enough anxiety to actually prevent some children from taking advantage of the aid. The second problem is that children are sometimes not given the training they need to use the aid effectively. A number of training programmes have been developed by educators which are designed to give the children the skills they need. These skills include looking and scanning techniques, recognizing appropriate materials to examine with the aid, correct posture, cleaning and maintenance. Acquisition of these skills will result in more efficient use (generally a higher speed while maintaining accuracy), and this, in turn, may result in more confidence in using the aid in public.

Closed circuit television (CCTV) is also used widely. This can help by enlarging print up to a size that is readable and it can also be used for diagrams. Reading speeds are often quite slow with a CCTV, and this can present a major problem in schools. Scanning diagrams needs considerable training, but, particularly with machines that have colour monitors, there is access to print and diagrams that might not otherwise be available. Unfortunately, if a machine is not available at home, or only available in one classroom, then its use may be a source more of frustration than of help to a child.

For some children, braille is the medium of communication. This code consists of about 150 shapes and over 250 rules of usage and so is not easy to learn. In addition, it is slow to read as only one shape can be perceived at a time, unlike print in which several words can be scanned in one glance. To help reading speed, the code uses a number of signs for common combinations of letters such as 'st', 'are' and 'tion' (see Fig. 11.1, p. 146). There are also abbreviations for some words, for example 'gd' for good, 'h' for have, 'brl' for braille.

Learning to read braille requires some 'pre-reading' activities as happens with print. Children who are sighted start reading after they have been exposed to print for several years in an informal way. Children need an equivalent experience of braille. They can begin to recognize patterns of braille dots as familiar words before starting formally to learn the alphabet. Many children in the preschool years follow a programme of tactile stimulation in which their fingers or, more accurately, their brains are trained to interpret tactile materials to prepare them to distinguish the small differences between braille letters.

Writing is usually carried out on a braille writing machine which has six keys, one for each dot in the braille 'cell'. As the process of learning braille is really the process of learning to read and write, many of the techniques used at the early stages are the same as used with print (*e.g.* writing short sentences, filling in missing words, labelling common objects).

Some children with very low levels of vision use both print and braille. Most often the combination is for children to read print with some form of aid and to write braille. Older children who can use a keyboard may type print, even though they need a CCTV or electronic speech output to read what they have written. More detail on the technology currently available to blind people can be found in Chapter 14.

These techniques and technology can help a child to function more efficiently. However, the psychological dilemma of working as both a blind and sighted person can create, at the least, some stress in the child. This may be particularly significant in the adolescent years when a child's self-concept may swing between being a very competent blind person to being a slow and inefficient sighted person.

There are a number of ways in which the classroom environment can be adapted to enable children with visual impairments to learn. Teachers need to consider the visual environment. The child should be seated where there is appropriate lighting. This may need to be at a higher or lower level of illumination depending on the eye defect. It may require the addition of a table lamp to illuminate a work surface or the use of blinds to control glare from outside. Glare, both direct from light sources and reflected off shiny surfaces, is the most common problem in the visual environment. Teachers need to provide appropriate contrast within the classroom to help the child locate furniture and obstacles around the room. High contrast is also needed on written material. Coloured pictures and print may need to be photocopied and important lines redrawn using a felt pen. Blackboard writing will be difficult to read unless the teacher makes a point of ensuring the board is really clean before use. Children may need to use black felt pens and write on lined paper.

Access to materials can also be assisted through the use of appropriate furniture. Children with poor vision often sit hunched over their desk, creating stress on their shoulders and backs and resulting in poor posture when sitting and standing. Desks with sloping tops and chairs carefully chosen for size can make a vast difference to such a child. These will enable them to work more comfortably and quickly with less tiredness over the day. Both blind and partially sighted children need extra space to store and arrange their books and equipment. The provision of extra large work surfaces and shelves can also make a considerable difference to efficiency and achievement.

Teachers will need to strive to provide the additional information needed by a child with visual impairments. Very often this will be given verbally, for example through descriptions of demonstrations, explanations of who has entered or left a room, and reasons for unexpected laughter. They may need to remember to read out what they write on a blackboard, or provide an individual copy of a handout that other children share. Several books are currently available which detail the techniques that can be used by class teachers to help a child with visual impairments learn with a mainstream class (*e.g.* Scholl 1986, Chapman and Stone 1988, Best 1992).

Inevitably there will be a number of subjects that create profound difficulties for a child with visual impairments. Experimental science and biology and physical education and games are often identified as creating special difficulties. If a child is to receive a satisfactory education, there needs to be a plan to give access to these important experiences. This is usually developed through discussion between the school and the visiting specialist teacher and may be provided through additional support staff at the school, special sessions outside the school day or even through schemes run by special schools during normal school holidays.

The special curriculum

Children with visual impairments will need some teaching on a special curriculum during their schooling. The central elements of this curriculum are listening skills, development of residual vision, social skills, orientation and mobility, activities of daily living, keyboard skills, use of drawings and signature writing.

Children with a visual impairment rely on auditory information more than other children. They need to learn to interpret sounds in the classroom as well as making sense of often incomplete verbal descriptions. Concentration on auditory information is tiring, and without being able to anticipate the onset of a sound, children often miss the beginning of a sentence.

All of these aspects of learning come under the heading of listening skills. Most children, but particularly those who lose their vision during school age, will need help to develop these skills to the high levels needed for efficient learning.

Activities of a teaching programme might be identifying sounds within a general hubbub of noise, identifying key phrases within a descriptive passage, following a series of spoken instructions, using a tape recorder for note taking.

Some children with low levels of vision can make better use of that vision if they are trained to use it. A number of training programmes have been developed in the USA and UK; most develop near vision for classroom tasks such as understanding diagrams and pictures. In these programmes, a series of test items assesses the use of visual and perceptual skills needed for these tasks such as the use of systematic scanning across a page, identifying a picture from its critical features, and familiarity with visual conventions of drawings and cartoons. A compensatory teaching programme will then be assembled and carried out to strengthen any areas of weakness. In mainstream schools, this will be the responsibility of specialist visiting teachers of the visually impaired. Timetabling these sessions is difficult and often involves taking a child out of class.

Both totally blind and low vision children can be taught mobility skills by the specialist teacher or by rehabilitation teachers trained specifically in this area. The skill of orientation is critical to efficient mobility. It refers to the ability to create mental maps of space and to understand one's position within the space. For example, very young blind babies are often observed to be confused when they roll over and find that the floor which was against their back is now 'above' them. Only with practice do they understand that it is they who move while the floor is fixed. Children standing up can often point to 'up' above their heads. But many blind children, while lying down, will still point (horizontally) above their heads when asked where 'up' is. Such children need additional practice to understand the concept of fixed reference points in space. They develop from an egocentric orientation, in which space is understood relative to their body, to a topographical model in which features in the physical surroundings provide the structure of space.

Many children, with some help, learn to find their way around familiar areas and make efficient use of tactile, auditory and visual clues. As they grow older and start to go about the neighbourhood on their own, they will need to develop skill in coping in unfamiliar surroundings, and this often requires the introduction of the long cane as an aid to mobility. This instruction often includes work in the child's home and neighbourhood as well as in school.

These examples of the special curriculum have been illustrated by reference to the children in a mainstream school. It must be remembered that more than half of all children with visual impairments have additional difficulties and that in a significant number of cases, children have severe learning difficulties (mental impairment). These children equally need access to a full curriculum and to the special curriculum. While the principles of their education are the same as those described above, teaching approaches and activities may be quite different. For example, areas of the special curriculum may be delivered through encouraging the child to reach for a sound-making toy using residual vision; providing contrasting tactile experiences such as warm, soapy and cold water; or placing the child on a wooden resonating board so that movement will be transmitted back to the child as vibration.

Conclusion

All children with visual impairments will need some help to access the full school curriculum. Technology can provide some of the support that is needed, but many difficulties arise from the restricted experiences available to children with visual impairments. To overcome these problems, children need access to informed teachers who can ensure they receive the compensatory experiences that will enable them to reach their true potential.

REFERENCES

Best, A.B. (1992) *Teaching Children with a Visual Impairment.* Milton Keynes: Open University Press.
Chapman, E.K., Stone, J. (1988) *The Visually Handicapped Child in Your Classroom.* London: Cassell.
Scholl, G.T. (1986) *The Foundations of Education for Blind and Visually Handicapped Children and Youth.* New York: American Foundation for the Blind.

14
THE CHALLENGE OF NEW TECHNOLOGY IN EDUCATION

Marianna Buultjens and Stuart Aitken

Although it is now more than a decade since the government initiative which provided at least one computer in every school in the UK, with similar developments occurring in many other industrialized countries, it is instructive that the adjective 'new' is still commonly used in educational circles when referring to computer/microelectronic technology. This may be related to the fact that the present majority of members of the teaching profession grew up without experiencing the benefits of this technology. It may also reflect the constant development in hardware and software applications which leaves many breathlessly trying to consolidate existing knowledge and skills while trying to keep up with the latest innovations. When asked 'What is the best computer to buy?', the reply is invariably 'The next one'.

Many developments in technology have been applied specifically to the blind or visually impaired. For instance, mobility aids have been designed which substitute aural or tactile signals for information normally detected through sight. Examples of the use of sound as a substitute for sight exist in the form of ultrasonic echo location devices such as the Sonicguide™ (Kay 1974); while the Mowatt Sensor employs touch to convey information on the proximity of obstacles in the blind person's environment. For the learner who is multiply disabled and blind or severely visually impaired, exciting possibilities are offered with the use of a 'Smart Wheelchair'. Through artificial speech it indicates to the user her/his approach to walls, door openings and other potential hazards (Nisbet 1989). To review the literature and issues raised by the application of these and other examples of compensatory technology would necessitate a wide-ranging discussion. However, in this chapter we will limit our consideration to the use of new technology within an educational context—school, college/university, home and to a lesser extent the workplace. Rather than mobility, we describe issues to do with information and communication.

Who faces the challenge?
Who then is facing the challenge of using technology within the curriculum and for gaining access to that curriculum? The list is long: teachers, therapists, advisory services, education consultants and teacher trainers; pupils and students who are blind or visually impaired and their families; commercial and non-commercial

hardware and software developers; schools, Local Education Authorities or State Departments of Education, voluntary and statutory bodies, and the legislative force of governments. It is not possible in the space of a short chapter to deal comprehensively with any one, let alone all, of these different groups and the implications of new technology for each. We intend to dedicate a section each to the challenges facing the teachers and those facing the pupils and students. By means of two short case studies we will then exemplify issues pertinent to the people and organizations mentioned above.

Challenges facing teachers

It is now accepted that information technology (IT) and microelectronic technology (MET) should form part of the range of methodologies employed by the class teacher in support of the different learning styles of pupils. Specialized switch inputs and interfaces can now operate battery toys, home electrical equipment such as television or radio (via a mains switcher[1]), music synthesisers (such as Smith Kettlewell's MIDI software, accessible to blind people, described by Heiner 1991) and computers. If used in a creative way with learners who are visually impaired/multiply disabled, motivation can be enhanced, sometimes indicating previously undetected learning potential (Bickerstaffe 1987, Pinkerton 1991, Aitken and Buultjens 1992).

The simple 'drill and practice' type of computer assisted instruction (CAI) software still has a limited place, while more in evidence are exploratory but fixed content programmes. Framework programmes, offering a template structure without specific content, allow teachers or pupils to define their own agenda and have led to more creative use of the computer. To customize these programmes for use by pupils who are visually impaired, teachers have to take into account factors such as screen colour and contrast, text size, and appropriateness of input through standard QWERTY keyboard, or adapted keyboard, braille keyboard or touch screen (Blenkhorn 1991, Painter 1991). Non-visual output can be provided by screen reading software linked to speech synthesizers, or in braille (in paper or electronic form).

The knowledge and skills demanded of the teacher are wide-ranging. S/he must not only understand the educational application of a wide range of equipment and software but also be experienced in the functional assessment of the needs of users (with or without multiple impairment). The task is daunting enough for the class teacher working in a special school for pupils who are blind or visually impaired, even more so for the teacher or lecturer in mainstream school or college who may have little access to specialist help.

More recent technologies which are now being promoted in schools in the UK, USA and elsewhere give access to much wider sources of information and learning.

---

[1]Mains switcher: a device which allows electrical appliances to be operated by an external switch, thus enabling severely disabled people to switch home appliances on and off.

CD-ROM[1] can offer local access to large databases and encyclopaedias and is being considered by education authorities as a potential alternative to the hard disk for storing collections of software, making these more accessible to schools. The take-up of Multimedia (its best known form currently being interactive video, IV[2]) has been relatively slow despite projects such as, in the UK, the BBC Domesday Project and the IVIS (Interactive Video in Schools) system. The high cost of equipment (although lower-cost packages are now available), coupled with its reliance on video and still images plus sound, has meant this medium has been largely overlooked by those working in the area of visual impairment. New editing software that allows for individual tailoring of activity, text/caption size, highlighting and zooming could open this valuable learning mechanism to partially-sighted users. However, CD-I[3], which is aimed at the consumer market and therefore benefits from economies of scale, may supersede IV as an educational and motivating tool for learners who are visually impaired.

From the list of equipment, software and applications it is clear that a teacher could profitably spend all her/his in-service training time developing skills in information technology. The National Curriculum of England and Wales encourages the use of IT through its cross-curricular status. The motivation and effort are not lacking. One only needs to consider the attendance at local or national exhibitions of educational technology such as BETT[4] to appreciate the level of interest. The problems are well recognized: lack of time for familiarization, lack of funds to acquire the equipment and programmes, and lack of both time and money to attend training courses.

Where such courses do exist and are accessible (*e.g.* short courses provided by educational consultants, the AFB[5] or RNIB[6], or modules forming part of specialist, award bearing courses for teachers of pupils with visual impairment), course organizers face a dilemma. On the one hand, they have to provide teachers with the opportunity to develop a breadth of knowledge, thereby enabling them to compare and evaluate across a range of products; on the other hand, time is needed to develop the necessary level of skills for confident and appropriate use of any single product. Figure 14.1 gives an idea of the scale and complexity of the task confronting educationists. It describes the broad categories of systems currently

---

[1]CD-ROM = compact disc, read-only memory, *i.e.* containing fixed information that cannot be altered by the user. It is an ideal medium for publishing large volumes of data cheaply. Text, graphics and sound are recorded on the disc digitally.

[2]IV combines the versatility of the microcomputer with the phenomenal video and digital storage capacity of the optical videodisc, which can hold approximately 155,000 analogue video images (pictures) on each side.

[3]CD-I = compact disc, interactive. A multimedia system for entertainment, education and information, it requires its own CD-I player (a computer in disguise). Sound, pictures, text and control software are all stored on the disc in digitized format. Audio and video can be combined for synchronized playback.

[4]BETT = British Educational Technology and Training—an exhibition bringing together commercial suppliers and educators. Similar large scale exhibitions take place annually in many other countries.

[5]AFB = American Federation for the Blind (New York, USA).

[6]RNIB = Royal National Institute for the Blind (London, UK).

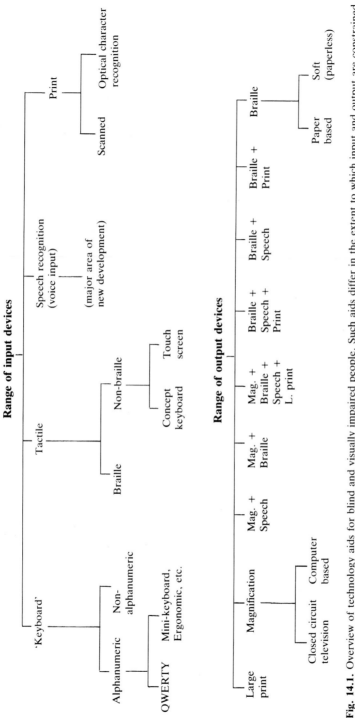

Fig. 14.1. Overview of technology aids for blind and visually impaired people. Such aids differ in the extent to which input and output are constrained. Each of the range of output categories is associated with many different types of devices, as exemplified in Figure 14.2.

166

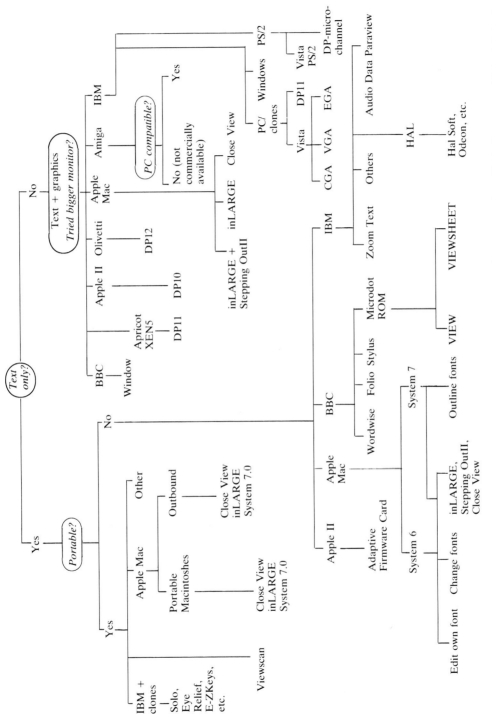

Fig. 14.2. Examples of computer based magnification aids for blind and visually impaired people. (The names of specific devices are provided solely to give an impression of the range of devices available.)

167

available, *e.g.* ones which operate by producing artificial speech, or ones in which text is inserted using an alphanumeric keyboard but where the output comes in the form of electronic or 'soft' braille. Figure 14.2 presents, in diagrammatic form, some of the options available within just one of these categories: computer based magnification systems. Any person familiar with the nightmare of customizing her/his own computer will appreciate the enormous problems of compatibility which may befall the less wary.

Challenges facing pupils at school

Over the past twenty years IT and MET, commencing with reading aids such as the Optacon (see p. 157), have greatly enhanced access to text based materials for learners who are blind or visually impaired. For instance, people who are partially sighted can now access enlarged materials in a variety of ways, augmenting the more traditional low vision aids: (i) stand-alone devices such as the ubiquitous closed circuit television; (ii) computer based magnification of text, or of text and graphics (the latter being essential for the student of statistics or for one who has to interpret diagrams or maps); (iii) more sophisticated means which act as screen reading software but, instead of producing artificial speech, produce enlarged text (this type of system is superior to simple magnification systems but carries a price: it entails more learning); (iv) most flexible of all, systems which allow the user to switch between artifical speech and enlarged text, with the press of a key. Which system is best? The answer will depend on the individual student and his or her stage of learning as well as the learning objectives in question. Figure 14.2 illustrates the wide range of computer based magnification systems available.

Screen reading applications with internal or external speech synthesizers have made word processing as accessible to blind users as to those with partial or normal sight. Even recent fears that graphical user interfaces (GUIs), such as those used with Apple Macintosh or Microsoft Windows, would cut off blind users from current and future developments have proved unfounded. Software developers have found ways of enabling blind users to enter and read text in this ultra-visual environment (Boyd *et al.* 1990). Nevertheless, very few devices have been designed solely with the needs of the blind person in mind. For the most part, standard computers are adapted via software and/or hardware to suit the needs of the blind or visually impaired person.

Case study

Rachel is 10 years old and totally blind from birth. She is multiply disabled, having cerebral palsy and no speech. Efforts had been made to try to teach her to sign; however, the lack of success resulted in questions being raised as to her general communicative ability. Intervention turned to the use of a portable communication aid which offers digitized speech. Real objects, associated with activities, were placed on top of 'squares' on the communication aid. When Rachel pressed the square a message was 'spoken'. This message had a strong association with the object. A start was made with one or two objects and messages, and these were then built upon. The most important questions for intervention centred on: choice of messages to be included; choice of objects to be associated with these messages; when objects should be changed so that more abstract forms of representation refer to the same spoken messages; which combinations of squares should be pressed in order to obtain messages; and whether one 'vocabulary set' should be arranged for home and another for school. Use of this communication aid revealed latent general communication abilities, and with it Rachel was able to make simple requests and demonstrate choice in her activities.

It has not, however, been a tale of unmitigated motivation and emancipation. Along with increased opportunities have come demands for additional and augmented skills not required to the same degree from the blind learner's peers—*e.g.* keyboarding and the ability to configure and then use a wide range of software, peripherals and different types of hardware. Trying to find time to fit this into a very full curriculum, in order to improve access to that curriculum, is a catch-22 situation faced by pupils/students and teachers alike.

Students in further or higher education
Several countries operate government schemes to assist disabled students in accessing materials through IT. For instance, in the UK an extension has been made to one government scheme: the Disabled Students Allowance. At the time of writing it offers £3000 for large items of equipment with an allowance of about £1000 per annum for smaller items. The money may be used to purchase equipment for college/university and home use. These sums can be augmented by as much as £4100 per annum to pay for readers, braille paper and other recurrent expenditure. Although this support is welcomed, it will not cover the costs of equipment for many blind students, who may require a computer, notetaker, cassette recorder, braille printer and scanner: this can easily total £10,000. Nor does money available from governments meet the actual costs involved for a disabled person. The following case study provides an illustration of the kind of equipment needs of higher education students.

Case study
John is a second year student at university, with severe visual impairment due to glaucoma. His initial request was for access to enlarging of screen information on a personal computer. An apparently simple request was complicated by the fact that, early on in the assessment, it was found that his course material would, in the following year, include a statistics package. Graphs and figures are an integral part of statistics. To provide access it is not possible to use software or hardware solutions which give only enlarging of characters. Because of the complexity of calculations which may be needed, it would be unlikely that any magnification which depends on accessing the computer's own 'working memory' would work: it would be too slow. A software solution was not really feasible, and a hardware solution was sought.

Although the request was for screen-based *magnification*, staff in a specialist assessment centre thought that he would benefit from the option of *speech synthesis* (though this would be of no use for presentation of graphs or figures). Ideally, he needed to switch immediately between magnification and speech synthesis. The computer needed to have enough ports to connect up to a printer, as well as to operate a mouse and a speech synthesizer. Even after delivery of the equipment, this very able student, already highly competent with technology, found that his system required modification so that it could be used with a particular type of monitor.

In the UK and elsewhere, no proportion of the award to a disabled student may be used to pay for assessment. Would you want to buy your medication from a pharmaceutical company? Unfortunately, there is no educational 'aspirin' for technology to be purchased over the counter.

In the workplace
In the UK, once in the workplace blind or visually impaired people will be helped to acquire necessary equipment by the Disablement Advisory Service and a Disablement Resettlement Officer. Similar schemes are operated in countries such as the USA, Canada, Sweden, Denmark and others. (The scheme is not limited to those who have come through further or higher education.) The importance of such schemes should not be underestimated. There are many disabled people working, and therefore paying taxes which quickly repay expenditure, who have been financed under this scheme. Leasing agreements ensure that equipment can be replaced when obsolete. Pockets of facilitative legislation do, therefore, currently exist, and if government departments could be organized around a structure which allowed liaison and cross-funding, the taxpayer would benefit enormously, wastage would be reduced and inefficiencies cut, and disabled people would have greater control over their own destiny. (For more comprehensive reading on computers at work and in daily life, see Davis 1991, Denton 1991, Hitchcock 1991, Sullivan 1991, Gill 1992.)

European Commission Directive 87/391
There is good news for all who use computers in the workplace (though some headaches for employers!) in this EC directive, which came into force at the end of 1992. Catching up with legislation in the USA, it recommends that employers: analyse the health and safety aspects of using workstations; provide training to employees before they start work on them; and consider issues of comfort and ease of use of equipment and software. Even more important, it stipulates that workers must be consulted and be able to participate in any matters covered by the directive. There will be implications in this directive, too, for education authorities and individual schools. Issues of health, safety, practicality and comfort will have to be considered for pupils, students and teachers.

At home
One issue often raised is that of 'high tech' in school or college but 'low tech' at home. Although using the most modern technology within the school environment, the pupil/student can be reduced to a state of dependence when it comes to reading

or writing if the same equipment is not available at home. What can be done to alleviate the school/home divide? There are two issues. One concerns the availability of equipment at home, while the second, often overlooked, is lack of technical support.

Availability of equipment at home

Several initiatives exist to assist in the purchase of technology for use by blind or visually impaired pupils. In the UK, these include a scheme run by the RNIB which part funds equipment used in a mainstream school. Joint schemes—wherein health authorities, education authorities and the social services contribute jointly to fund equipment—can ensure a higher degree of continuity between school and home. These initiatives, coupled with leasing schemes, could reduce significantly the degree of uncertainty experienced by pupils and parents. It is not difficult to imagine how such a scheme could be extended across regional or state boundaries. This would eradicate the problem of parents having to begin funding efforts all over again when moving home out of one region or state to another. A scheme may exist already in the workplace; for instance, the aforementioned Disablement Advisory Service will fund equipment for people who are registered disabled.

Technical support

Provision of equipment is only one aspect of *using* that equipment. If teachers experience difficulties in the technological jungle, what about parents and pupils themselves? At home there will not be the same recourse to a school's technician and computing teacher. Vincent (1991) elucidated several simple solutions to this pressing problem. He stressed the importance of allowing a gradual progression in the complexity of equipment used. By judicious choice of a couple of computer games, the blind pupil may thereby enlist the willing services of a neighbour or relative who is close to hand. In addition, blind and visually impaired people themselves have formed special interest groups covering several specific areas of technology.

Conclusion

Within barely a decade we have moved from the excitement of the first Apple II or BBC computers arriving in USA and UK schools, respectively, to the recent news that 'virtual reality' is in the curriculum for High Schools in Ontario, Canada (Sherman 1992). Technology has liberated many severely disabled people and let them show how they communicate, learn, contribute to and enrich the quality of our society. The challenge for us all is to be receptive, perceptive and determined, and to keep technology 'working' for pupils and students.

REFERENCES

Aitken, S., Buultjens, M. (1992) *Vision for Doing: Assessing Functional Vision of Learners Who Are*

Multiply Disabled. Edinburgh: Moray House.

Bickerstaffe, A. (1987) 'A new approach to special care.' *Talking Sense*, **33**, 6–7.

Blenkhorn, P. (1991) 'Computer technology: developments to come.' *Eye Contact*, **1**, 25–26.

Boyd, L.H., Boyd, W.L., Vanderheiden, G.C. (1990) 'The Graphical User Interface: crisis, danger and opportunity.' *Journal of Visual Impairment and Blindness*, **84**, 496–502.

Davis, N. (1991) 'Computers at work: synthetic speech systems.' *The New Beacon*, **75**, (887), 202–204.

Denton, B. (1991) 'Computers at work: enhanced character systems.' *The New Beacon*, **75**, (885), 110–114.

Gill, J.M. (1992) 'Technology in the 1990s: some European initiatives.' *The New Beacon*, **76**, (895), 45–59.

Heiner, D. (1991) 'RESNA '91: Technology for the Nineties: A personal account' *Communication Outlook*, **13**, 4–8.

Hitchcock, S. (1991) 'Computers at work: electronic braille systems.' *The New Beacon*, **75**, (889), 282–284.

Kay, L. (1974) 'Orientation for blind persons: clear path indicator or environmental sensor.' *New Outlook for the Blind*, **68**, 289–296.

Nisbet, P. (1989) 'The Smart Wheelchair.' *In:* Korba, L.W. (Ed.) *International Inventory of Robotics Projects in the Health Care Field.* Ottowa: National Research Council.

Painter, C. (1991) 'Computer technology: developments to date.' *Eye Contact*, **1**, 15–16.

Pinkerton, S. (1991) 'Active learning through the use of microtechnology.' *In:* Watson, J. (Ed.) *Innovatory Practice and Severe Learning Difficulties.* Edinburgh: Moray House, pp. 1–12.

Sherman, B. (1992) 'Birth of a brave new world.' *The Times Educational Supplement, Computer Update* (March), p. 3.

Sullivan, D. (1991) 'Computers at work: making computers work for you.' *The New Beacon*, **75**, (883), 9–13.

Vincent, T.V. (1991) 'The role of technology in distance education: some experiences at the Open University.' *In:* Buultjens, M., Baikie, R. (Eds) *Scottish Education for the Nineties: Learning with Visual Impairment.* Edinburgh: Moray House, p. 91.

15
SOCIAL ASPECTS OF VISUAL IMPAIRMENT

Robert Greenhalgh

Historically, at least in the UK, workers in the social services have not played a major part in the management of the visually impaired child, nor have they been closely involved in the problems encountered by the family. It has been assumed that any problems would be dealt with by the health or educational services. The assumption has been that there is little need for social service involvement until the child reaches adulthood. Clearly, this is unreasonable in today's climate where the range of problems encountered by the child and the family is becoming increasingly complex.

There is a need for the whole family to have a single worker who can be contacted as their advocate and who can facilitate the decision making process for them. The decisions they are likely to have to make will involve educational, health and social issues. Families with normally sighted children do not have to make these decisions or deal with the bureaucracy surrounding the service network. Certainly, they have to address educational, health and social issues, but in the context of decisions which will be made by the majority of people in their community. The family of the visually impaired child has to make these decisions without peer support. A comprehensive multidisciplinary approach can provide the solution.

The role of the social worker

One of the primary reasons for there being a lack of contact between the social services and the visually impaired child was that most of the children would be placed in special schools for the visually impaired, often many miles from home, which necessitated residential education. There were, of course, some day schools, but these were not available in every area.

The special schools were expected to look after the needs of the child, but little if any attention was given to the needs of the family. The child's residence in school meant that the family would only have contact during holidays. Frequently there would be changes in the child's behaviour, maturity and skills during the term. In consequence the family would welcome a 'stranger' when holiday time arrived. The child would have little in common with other children in the home area and thus would be more 'at home' at school. Occasionally, social service workers would make efforts to cater for the needs of the child during holidays, but this would generally be within a group of other visually impaired children from the area. This added to the child's isolation from peers in the home community.

The more recent trend to adopt integrated rather than segregated schooling has changed the strategies of social service workers and has created problems for the 'caring system' which were not originally envisaged. For example, the special schools have found that their facilities are too large for the population of children who now require to attend them and as a result they have had to diversify by considering provision for further education and prevocational studies. Unfortunately, there has also been a tendency for schools to enter into competition for the reduced population of visually impaired children eligible for their services.

The social services worker, usually a rehabilitation worker for the visually impaired, is likely to have contact with a visually impaired person from birth until death whenever there is a problem related to that visual impairment. The rehabilitation worker is therefore ideally placed to undertake two roles. The first is that of advocate for the family. In this role the worker can help the family to understand the options which are available to them in determining the best route through the educational system for their child. The family has to come into contact with a range of professionals from a number of different disciplines during the child's educational years, and the presence of a stable and constant figure who represents their particular needs is essential.

The rehabilitation worker can work with the child and the family during the preschool years, when part of the task may be to help the family to come to terms with the emotional crises involved in them having a disabled child. S/he can then help to prepare the child and the family for education, and later can help them to move through the change from school to further education, vocational training, or employment. Specialists in education, training or employment (or unemployment!) are likely to be involved at the same time; however, it is the independence of the rehabilitation worker which the parents require in order to ensure that there is objectivity and impartiality in the decision making process.

Specialists in education and employment may, understandably, have a bias toward a particular style of education or a particular kind of training or employment. The danger is that this bias may be toward the more traditional solutions rather than solutions which are in the best developmental interests of the child. For example, there is still a tendency to consider employment in terms of 'what a visually impaired person can do' rather than considering what the individual wants to do and then determining whether this is possible and what adaptations would be required in the light of the impairment.

The second role is that of 'key-worker'. The multiplicity of disciplines involved with the visually impaired child and the family requires coordination. There is likely to be contact with an ophthalmologist, an optometrist, a paediatrician, a general practitioner, an educational psychologist, a peripatetic teacher, a community nurse, an employment advisor, an orthoptist, a rehabilitation worker and so on. Often there is little real liaison between these professionals, and help and advice are given in isolation. This seems to be unwise, as inter- and multi-disciplinarity can combine to produce the most effective and realistic solutions.

Some of the professionals will only see the child on occasions, and some may never actually see the whole family. The key worker can ensure that professionals are brought together at the right time, that the parents and the child are involved at appropriate times and that the parents are fully informed about their child's situation throughout.

The rehabilitation worker must retain contact with the child whether education is in a special school or in an integrated setting. In either case it is undoubtedly her/his responsibility to ensure that the child is integrated into the community. There is also a need for family support to help the parents understand what is happening to their child, and also to help maintain a balance when there are other children in the family. Siblings can over-protect, be jealous of the attention received by the visually impaired child, use the visually impaired child as a scapegoat in the presence of friends, and so on. It is the role of the rehabilitation worker to facilitate the understanding of all the members of the family so that it remains a coherent and balanced whole.

Involving the child in activities within the home community needs careful thought and preparation. For example, if the child is to be introduced to a local scout group or fishing club then the existing members of the group need to be prepared with the knowledge and skills so that the visually impaired child can be assimilated into the group with the minimum of difficulty and potential embarrassment. This is the function of the rehabilitation worker.

The rehabilitation worker can play an important part in the process of assessment, which must be reviewed and repeated at regular intervals. Assessment needs to be comprehensive, examining the child's sensory, physical and intellectual abilities and disabilities. This is particularly important in the growing group of children who have additional disabilities.

This brief discussion of the role of the social services indicates how important it is that rehabilitation workers receive appropriate training about the visually impaired child, understanding the roles and responsibilities of other professionals involved with the child and family, appreciating the limits of the social service role, and representing the interests of the child and family.

Functionally sighted or functionally blind?

Rehabilitation workers are increasingly being trained to work on vision enhancement techniques with all of their visually impaired clients who show some sign of being functionally sighted. Today, many professionals from many disciplines are enthusiastic and excited about the development of visual skills. However, in the case of the visually impaired child we have to keep such skills within a realistic perspective.

Children, like any other age group of visually impaired people, are likely to use one of three different coping strategies for acquiring information. Effective information gathering is vital if the child is to be given the maximum opportunity of developing her/his intellectual and emotional potential. These three coping strategies are: (i) to use vision as the primary sense for gathering information and for directing behaviour; (ii) to use the non-visual senses for gathering information and for directing behaviour; and (iii) to use vision in some circumstances and the non-visual senses in others.

Whether the child is in a special school or an integrated educational setting there will be a need for some assistance in helping to develop the appropriate strategy. This is an area where the rehabilitation worker can complement work undertaken in the school. It is important that there is consistency between the encouragement given at school and that given at home. The child should be consistently encouraged to develop the most appropriate strategies.

The difficulty arises within the strategy which requires the child to use the visual and the non-visual senses situationally. This can be confusing for the child, and a preference for using either the visual or the non-visual senses can develop. It is thus important that the child's behaviour is reinforced appropriately so that information gathering is maximized.

There are still occasions when children are encouraged to use braille as a method of reading and writing when print reading would be both possible and practical. This practice tends to limit the child's exposure to information because, contrary to popular opinion, it is not a natural feature of behaviour to seek appropriate visual stimulation. Parents and children are unlikely to question the decision of a school which recommends the use of braille as opposed to print. Perhaps there is still some of the philosophy of sight saving within our professions? Maybe some of us still hang on to the concept of 'training to be blind' or 'preparing for blindness'. There is no preparation for blindness, it must be dealt with when it occurs. Experience tells us time and time again that people who are taught sight saving techniques while they still have some sight will need retraining when sight is eventually lost.

The rehabilitation worker can help the child to develop non-visual skills, can help the child to develop sight enhancement strategies, can help to train the child to use a range of aids to vision. More importantly, the rehabilitation worker can help the family to understand and use these strategies and techniques so that they become an acceptable part of everyday life.

Frequently the child's home will not be designed to maximize visual potential, and this will include the child's own room within the home. Families need to be aware of the need for the appropriate use of light, contrast and size in creating a visual environment which will allow the child to function comfortably using any available vision. People need to be made aware of the benefits of manipulating these three crucial variables of vision. We do not always use common sense in creating the visual environment within which we live. The indoor environment can be controlled cheaply and effectively.

Of course, the same principles apply to schools as well as private houses. I suspect that some salutary lessons could be learned if school staff carried out an audit of their visual environments. The colour of the walls, the positioning of

176

machines like closed circuit television (CCTV) systems, the marking of routes around the school, the amenity lighting around the outside of the buildings, and so on.

Teachers in integrated educational settings may well require more help than their colleagues in special schools. I can recall being consulted by the parents of a 12-year-old girl who was placed in a large comprehensive school. Undoubtedly the child could cope within the setting with some specialized help and equipment. The school helped acquire a CCTV system which could be moved from class to class without a great deal of difficulty. Unfortunately, neither teachers nor parents knew very much about CCTVs. The objective when the system was purchased was to help the girl to lead a normal life within the school and feel a part of her peer group in classes. The CCTV was placed 15cm from the blackboard, about 1.25m in front of the nearest member of the class! This exaggerated rather than eradicated the differentness of the girl. Once the CCTV was set up in a more appropriate part of the classroom, and the pupil, teacher and other class members were informed about what it was and what it could do, there was a different atmosphere within the classroom.

The philosophy of moving from segregated to integrated education is admirable, but must be thoroughly thought through and adequately resourced. The institutionalizing philosophies of the segregated schooling system must be eradicated because they lead to stereotyped visually impaired individuals entering society at a disadvantage when they reach the age at which they need vocational training or employment. At this stage it is often too late for the rehabilitation worker to 'socialize' the person: the socializing damage has been done within the special education system.

The rehabilitation worker can help with advice in integrated education settings about how to provide an appropriate visual environment for visually impaired pupils. This advice is not always available through the peripatetic teacher. Again this directs us toward a multidisciplinary approach through the professional services of a 'vision team'.

The vision team
Expertise in education, social work and employment varies enormously from country to country and from area to area. There are examples of parents moving house to a completely new area in order to take advantage of particular educational or social service facilities. We have to maximize all of our professional strengths and resources for the effective management of the visually impaired child. This might mean moving across traditional geographical and disciplinary boundaries, a movement which workers are reticent to make and which the various bureaucracies involved with service control are loath to accept. However, we must service the 'whole family' ideal with a 'whole system' approach.

This indicates the need for a vision team. The vision team need not be based in the same geographical location nor do all the members of that team need to have frequent contact with each other. The word 'team' is used loosely to point out that each member has a part to play in the development of the visually impaired child and may need to be brought in for discussion and assistance at critical points in the developmental process.

Team members will include professionals from the 'health' professions such as the ophthalmologist, the optometrist, the orthoptist, the general practitioner and the community nurse. Their function will be to consider the pathology and maximize the child's physical abilities. There is likely to be a need for a lot of contact in the initial stages of assessment, because assessment must be both clinical and functional. It is the marriage of the two techniques which brings realistic solutions to the child's potential problems. These workers may be required for advice and further assessment later in the child's career.

Clearly, it is essential that educationalists are a part of the team as they can help to provide solutions to the child's learning problems.

Employment specialists need to be included as it is important that career prospects are kept under review from an early stage. The transition from school to further education, vocational training or employment is a critical stage in an individual's life and it must be thoroughly thought through. The young person must learn that s/he is an individual in an adult world and that s/he has responsibilities for her/himself. A service system is there to assist, not to direct or to take over the decision making process. Unfortunately there is still a tendency for people to become a part of the 'visual handicap' system and be 'processed' by that system much to the detriment of the process of 'normalization'.

I believe that the rehabilitation worker should be the key worker within the vision team. This worker should be responsible for calling case conferences and ensuring that all the relevant members of the team are in contact with each other and are updated on the child's progress. Appropriate disciplines or people from a mix of disciplines should be called in to resolve particular problems.

My discussion of the professionals involved in the vision team is not meant to be complete. I am simply presenting a case for collaboration and cooperation in the interests of the community. There must be other disciplines involved, but space does not allow for an exhaustive examination.

This sounds complex. I do not think that it is, it is merely a systematic and efficient way of helping a visually impaired child and her/his family to cope with a range of problems and difficulties which are likely to be alien to them.

The model of management which I am suggesting requires that people within the relevant disciplines remove some defensiveness from their approach to their own skills and knowledge. We can provide a much more holistic and appropriate service if we have more appreciation of the limits and boundaries of all of the professionals involved in the process. Particularly, we should not be threatened by the concept of moving closer to other professionals and being involved with them in an attempt to enrich what is already a well developed service.

It is often helpful to consider the nature of practice in other countries in developing a 'home' strategy. However, there is no easy comparison in this case. Other European countries, for instance, have tended to develop their system of care very differently to that in the UK. Although it is possible to examine the educational system, or the social service system or the health care system of other countries in isolation, my experience does not allow me to offer a useful comparison of the holistic approach which I am advocating. Models of care do not transfer well from one country to another, or from one culture to another. It is better to examine a number of different models of service and produce one which combines elements of many but which is appropriate for the country and culture in which it is to operate.

Conclusion

There is a need for a continuous process of assessment, education, counselling and advice throughout the visually impaired child's life. We need to involve a range of disciplines in a systematic way and ensure that the child's family and home community are properly involved in the whole process.

I suggest that, as with sighted children as they grow older, there is a need to pass responsibility from the family and the visual disability service system back to the child who must become a fully functioning adult in a complex and sometimes hostile society.

16
PREVENTION OF CHILDHOOD BLINDNESS

Clare Gilbert

Magnitude of childhood blindness

Sources of prevalence data include population based surveys and blind person registers. Table 16.1 summarizes available data from these sources.

These figures are likely to underestimate the true figure for a variety of reasons. Blind person registers are usually voluntary and do not include all children eligible for registration (Goggin and O'Keefe 1991). Population based surveys do not take into account children in schools for the blind, and due to difficulties in measuring visual acuity in young children, those with visual loss but without obvious ocular abnormalities may be missed (Chirambo *et al.* 1986).

Using the limited data that are available it is estimated that there are around 1.5 million blind children in the world, 85 per cent of whom live in Africa and Asia (WHO 1992) (Table 16.2).

Accurate incidence data are not available but it is estimated that 500,000 children become blind each year (WHO 1992). Many of the blinding conditions of childhood in developing countries are associated with a high mortality rate, *i.e.* measles infection, vitamin A deficiency and congenitally acquired rubella. It is thought that 60 to 80 per cent of children die within one to two years of becoming blind (Cohen *et al.* 1985).

Major causes of childhood blindness

Data on causes of blindness in children come from blind person registers, and from blind school and hospital based studies. Comparing data from these sources is difficult, as different definitions and classification systems have been used. It is possible, however, to recategorize and analyse the data using a descriptive, anatomical classification. Recently a form for recording causes of blindness and visual loss has been developed in order to provide a standardized methodology (Gilbert 1993*b*).

Causes of visual loss can be classified anatomically or aetiologically. An anatomical classification is useful for situations where medical records or details of past medical history are absent or scanty, as the site of abnormality leading to visual loss can be determined by clinical examination.

Anatomical classification

Table 16.3 summarizes data from blind school and hospital based studies, and information obtained from blind person registers (Foster 1988).

TABLE 16.1

Prevalence data on childhood blindness

Country (Reference)	Year of study	Prevalence/1000	Source of data
England (RNIB 1985)	1985	0.10 (0–4 yrs) 0.22 (5–9 yrs) 0.23 (10–14 yrs)	Registration
Eire (Goggin and O'Keefe 1991)	1991	0.20 (0–16 yrs)	Estimate from identified children
Scandinavia (Riise et al. 1992)	1992	0.15–0.41	Registration
Iceland (Halldorsson and Bjornsson 1980)	1980	0.36 (10–14 yrs)	Survey
UK (Stewart-Brown 1988)	1988	0.34 (10 yrs)	Cohort study
Nepal (Brilliant 1988)	1981	0.63 (0–14 yrs)	Survey
Bangladesh (Cohen et al. 1985)	1983	0.64 (0–5 yrs rural) 1.09 (0–5 yrs urban)	Survey
Malawi (Chirambo 1986)	1986	1.10 (0–5 yrs)	Survey
The Gambia (Faal 1989)	1986	0.7 (0–19 yrs)	Survey
Benin (WHO 1991)	1991	0.6 (0–15 yrs)	Survey

TABLE 16.2

Estimated prevalence of childhood blindness, by region*

Region	Under-16 population (millions)	Blindness prevalence (per 1000)	Estimated no. of blind children
Africa	240	1.1	264,000
Asia	1200	0.9	1,080,000
Latin America	130	0.6	78,000
Europe/USA/Japan	240	0.3	72,000

*WHO (1992).

There is marked regional variation, with corneal disease (mainly scarring and phthisis bulbi) being the most common cause of childhood blindness in Africa and southern Asia. Conditions of the retina (mainly dystrophies) and of the optic nerve and higher visual pathways are more important causes in industrialized countries.

181

TABLE 16.3
Anatomical causes of childhood blindness, by region*

Region	E. Africa (N=1845) %	W. Africa (N=567) %	S. Asia (N=424) %	L. America (N=991) %	Europe/USA (N=1806) %
Cornea/phthisis	72	39	33	8	1
Lens	6	15	7	20	8
Uvea	2	6	1	1	1
Retina	3	11	20	26	30
Glaucoma	1	10	5	10	2
Optic nerve	6	7	5	10	23
Other	10	12	29	25	35

*Foster (1988)

Given a prevalence of 1.5 million blind children and the relative importance of the various anatomical causes of blindness as determined in different parts of the world, it is possible to make some crude estimates of the magnitude of childhood blindness associated with each of the various anatomical sites. These estimates are presented in Tables 16.4 and 16.5.

Aetiological classification
The aetiological classification employs the time of onset of the insult that led to blindness, as follows.
(1) Factors operating at conception:
   —genetic disease;
   —chromosomal abnormalities.
(2) Factors operating during the intrauterine period:
   —intrauterine infection, *e.g.* rubella;
   —toxins, *e.g.* alcohol, drugs.
(3) Factors operating during the perinatal and neonatal period:
   —birth trauma;
   —preterm birth, *e.g.* retinopathy of prematurity (ROP);
   —infection, *e.g.* ophthalmia neonatorum.
(4) Factors operating during infancy and childhood:
   —vitamin A deficiency (VAD);
   —measles;
   —trauma.
(5) Unclassifiable: this includes conditions, often present since birth, where the underlying cause is not known and where the abnormality cannot be attributed to genetic disease or events occurring during the intrauterine period.
   Few aetiological data are available. Table 16.6 summarizes data from blind school studies undertaken in West Africa, South India and Chile (Gilbert *et al.* 1993*a*).

TABLE 16.4

Prevalence of childhood blindness from corneal scarring and phthisis bulbi

Socioeconomic status	Example countries	Corneal scar/phthisis	Est. no. blind	Est. no. blind from corneal scar/phthisis
Very low	Ethiopia Malawi	65–75%	350,000	227,500–262,500
Low	India Ghana	35–45%	613,000	215,000–276,000
Moderate	Peru Chile	5–10%	424,000	21,000–42,000
Good	USA UK	0–1%	63,000	0–600

TABLE 16.5

Estimated numbers of blind children worldwide, by anatomical cause

Corneal scarring/phthisis bulbi	500,000
Cataract	200,000
Retina	300,000
Optic nerve	100,000
Glaucoma	100,000
Other	300,000
Total	1,500,000

TABLE 16.6

Aetiological classification of childhood blindness, by region*

Aetiology	W. Africa (N=284) %	S. India (N=305) %	Chile (N=217) %
Hereditary	21	30	30
Intrauterine	8	1	9
Perinatal	2	2	21
Childhood	34	37	12
Unclassified	35	30	28

*Gilbert *et al.* (1993*a*)

In countries with severely limited health services and resources, factors operating during childhood, mainly vitamin A deficiency and measles, account for the highest proportion of blindness in children. Perinatal factors become more important in countries with moderately developed health care services, *e.g.* Chile, where ROP is an emerging problem. In Europe and North America, genetic disease accounts for approximately 50 per cent of childhood blindness (Jay 1987,

Rosenberg *et al.* 1992), reflecting high levels of socioeconomic development and good health care provision.

Principles of prevention

The term 'prevention' can be thought of as having four components when used in the context of visual loss or disability.

(1) Primary prevention (prevention of the disease):
   —health promotion;
   —health education;
   —primary health care programmes.
(2) Secondary prevention (to prevent visual loss from established disease):
   —early identification of cases;
   —appropriate treatment and management.
(3) Tertiary prevention (to restore visual function in blind or severely visually impaired people).
(4) Prevention of disability by:
   —special education;
   —rehabilitation;
   —vocational training.

These principles form a useful framework when considering the control of blindness in children.

Blindness from corneal scarring

In developing countries corneal scarring usually results from a complex interaction of different mechanisms including VAD, measles, herpes simplex keratitis and the use of harmful traditional eye medicines and ocular practices. VAD is the single most important factor, accounting for an estimated 40 to 50 per cent of childhood blindness worldwide. Ophthalmia neonatorum, trauma and infective corneal ulceration are other causes of corneal scarring.

Vitamin A deficiency

Vitamin A is found as retinol in animal food sources, *e.g.* breast milk, cheese, fish, liver and eggs, and as carotenes and carotenoids in plant sources, *e.g.* certain fruits (mango, papaya), dark green leafy vegetables and red palm oil. Vitamin A is necessary for cell differentiation and growth, particularly of epithelial tissues, and is an essential component of photoreceptor visual pigment (rhodopsin). Vitamin A also plays a role in the immune system (Ross 1992). 95 per cent of total body vitamin A is stored in the liver as retinal palmitate, and stores are usually sufficient for 6 months. Vitamin A is released from the liver bound to retinol binding protein, which is transported to tissues bound to pre-albumin.

VAD usually results from a combination of poor dietary intake, malabsorption and increased tissue demand. It is a condition of poverty, reflecting low levels of socioeconomic development and education, and poor health care provision. Low

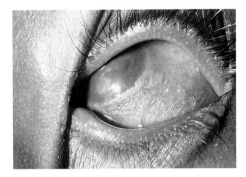

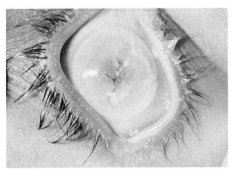

Fig. 16.1. Xerophthalmia in a girl from Nepal, showing corneal and conjunctival xerosis (X1A, X2) and a Bitot's spot (X1B).

Fig. 16.2. Corneal necrosis (keratomalacia, X3B) caused by vitamin A deficiency.

dietary intake does not necessarily mean that affordable vitamin A rich foods are not available; inadequate breast feeding, traditional weaning and child feeding practices and taboos are also important factors. VAD is often associated with protein energy malnutrition and deficiency of other micronutrients. Severe diarrhoea is a cause of malabsorption, and measles infection leads to increased demand for vitamin A. Children born in communities where women of child-bearing age have low vitamin A levels are also more likely to be deficient (Fairney *et al.* 1987). Children who are already vitamin A deficient with reduced liver stores can be precipitated into acute deficiency by measles infection or severe diarrhoea, resulting in xerophthalmia and nutritional blindness.

In VAD dedifferentiation of conjunctival and corneal epithelium leads to loss of goblet cells, squamous metaplasia and xerosis of the conjunctiva and cornea (xerophthalmia). Bacterial action on deposits of keratin in the conjunctiva leads to accumulation of material which has a white, foamy, cottage-cheese like appearance. These accumulations, Bitot's spots, are usually located temporally (Fig. 16.1). Acute VAD can lead to corneal ulceration and necrosis (keratomalacia) (Fig. 16.2). Reduced photoreceptor rhodopsin causes night blindness and, in advanced cases, an abnormal fundus appearance.

A grading system for xerophthalmia has been developed by the World Health Organization (1982) (Table 16.7).

Conjunctival xerosis and Bitot's spots are a sign of long-standing VAD, found principally in children aged 3 to 8 years. Children most at risk of keratomalacia and blindness are those aged 6 months to 4 years, who may not have exhibited the other features of xerophthalmia before the onset of corneal ulceration (Sommer 1982). For this reason it is important to be able to identify *communities* at risk of VAD as well as individual children.

The association between VAD and blindness has been known for a long time. Recent population based intervention studies have clearly demonstrated that VAD

185

TABLE 16.7

Grading of xerophthalmia*

Conjunctival xerosis	X1A
Bitot's spots with conjunctival xerosis	X1B
Corneal xerosis	X2
Corneal ulceration <1/3 of cornea	X3A
Corneal ulceration ≥1/3 of cornea	X3B
Night blindness	XN
Xerophthalmic fundus	XF
Corneal scar	XS

*WHO (1982).

is also associated with increased mortality (Sommer *et al.* 1986, Ramatullah *et al.* 1990, Vijayaraghavan *et al.* 1990, West *et al.* 1991, Daulaire *et al.* 1992). Identification of an individual child with VAD, and of communities of children at risk, is therefore important not only to prevent blindness but also for child survival.

ASSESSMENT OF VITAMIN A DEFICIENCY

VAD in *individual children* can be assessed (i) biochemically, by measuring serum retinol levels (normal >200μg/L), or by assessing liver stores using the relative dose response or the modified relative dose response; (ii) histologically, using conjunctival impression cytology (CIC); and (iii) clinically, by ocular examination for signs of xerophthalmia. Each of these methods has limitations if used in isolation: blood tests because there is seasonal variation in serum vitamin A levels; CIC because of difficulty in obtaining good samples from young children and in interpreting borderline changes; and clinical signs because not all those who are vitamin A deficient using other criteria show signs of xerophthalmia.

For planning health care programmes it is important to identify communities of children at risk so that they can be targeted with vitamin A programmes. A simple, quick and cheap way of assessing the vitamin A status of a community is to determine the prevalence of xerophthalmia, particularly of Bitot's spots. The World Health Organization (1982) suggested minimal prevalence criteria for the different grades of xerophthalmia to indicate areas where there is a significant public health problem (Table 16.8). The prevalence of any condition is a reflection of the incidence and duration of the condition, either to resolution of disease or death of the individual. The level of corneal xerosis/ulceration that is considered significant is low because these conditions are transient, with resolution to corneal scarring or because the child subsequently dies.

Children with xerophthalmia represent only the 'tip of the iceberg' of those who are deficient in vitamin A in the community; the specificity and sensitivity of some of the methods outlined above, *e.g.* CIC, are being evaluated as ways of detecting subclinical deficiency (Gadomski *et al.* 1989, Reddy *et al.* 1989). A combination of tests may prove to be the best way of assessing vitamin A status in

TABLE 16.8

Public health significance of xerophthalmia: minimal prevalence criteria*

Grade		Minimal prevalence /10,000 children
XN	Night blindness	100
X1B	Bitot's spots	50
X2, X3A, X3B	Corneal xerosis/ulcer	5
XS	Corneal scar	10

*WHO (1982).

individuals and communities under the varied conditions commonly associated with VAD (Underwood 1990*a*).

PREVENTIVE STRATEGIES

The long-term solution to VAD lies in improving the health and nutrition of preschool children through health promotion and socioeconomic development in at-risk communities. In the short term, sustainable vitamin A supplementation programmes and treatment of individual children at risk are indicated in areas where VAD is a public health problem (Underwood 1990*b*).

(1) Primary prevention (prevention of VAD: improve intake of vitamin A in children and in women of child-bearing age; prevent malabsorption; prevent measles):

—health promotion, *e.g.* breast feeding;

—health and nutrition education;

—promote home gardening;

—vitamin A fortification of commonly consumed foods;

—diarrhoea control and oral rehydration therapy;

—measles immunization programmes;

—vitamin A prophylaxis of individual children at risk, *i.e.* those with measles and severe diarrhoea from communities at risk (Table 16.9);

—mass distribution of vitamin A to communities at risk (Table 16.10).

(2) Secondary prevention (prevention of blindness in children with xerophthalmia:

—vitamin A treatment for all children with signs of xerophthalmia (Table 16.9).

(3) Tertiary prevention (restoration of sight in children with corneal scarring):

—optical iridectomy for central corneal scars;

—corneal grafting (only recommended for situations with good ophthalmic facilities and where follow-up can be guaranteed).

Measles

Measles infection is a leading cause of child mortality in developing countries,

TABLE 16.9

Treatment schedule for children with xerophthalmia and for those with measles or severe diarrhoea from communities at risk*

	Children <12 months	Children >12 months
Day 1	100,000 IU orally or 50,000 IU i.m.	200,000 IU orally or 100,000 IU i.m.
Day 2	Repeat	Repeat
Day 3	Repeat	Repeat

*Sommer (1982).

TABLE 16.10

Vitamin A schedules for community treatment

Children <12 months	100,000 IU—every 4–6 mths
Children > 12 months	200,000 IU—every 4–6 mths
Neonate[1]	50,000 IU—at birth
Mothers post partum	300,000 IU—within 1 mth of delivery
Pregnant[2] and lactating[1] women	5,000 IU—daily
	or
	20,000 IU—weekly

[1]Lower doses are required as high doses are toxic to neonates.
[2]Lower doses should be given during pregnancy because of possible teratogenic effects (Nelson 1990).

accounting for an estimated 1.5 million deaths per year (Henderson *et al.* 1988). The case fatality rate is much higher in developing than in industrialized countries (Aaby 1988), particularly in children aged 4 to 12 months (Garenne *et al.* 1991). Measles infection is rare in children under the age of 4 months due to the protective effect of maternal antibodies.

Hospital based studies in Africa have shown that corneal ulceration followed measles infection in 0.75 to 3.3 per cent of cases (Morley *et al.* 1967, Kimati and Lyaruu 1976, Animashaun 1977, Pepping *et al.* 1987). Blind school studies have indicated that up to 81 per cent of cases of corneal scarring followed measles infection (Sandford-Smith and Whittle 1979), while hospital based studies of children with corneal ulceration revealed that measles infection preceded the ulcer in 36 per cent of cases (Foster and Sommer 1986).

The pathogenesis of corneal scarring following measles infection is complex and multifactorial. The following mechanisms have been implicated: acute VAD leading to keratomalacia; secondary herpes simplex virus (HSV) keratitis; secondary bacterial infection; exposure keratitis; and the use of traditional eye medicines. In a study of 48 Tanzanian children with corneal ulceration following measles infection 24 had keratomalacia, 10 HSV keratitis and six measles keratitis, while in eight the ulceration was attributed to the use of traditional medicines

(Foster and Sommer 1986).

Children with measles infection have lower serum vitamin A levels than age/sex matched controls. Reduced intake, malabsorption, protein losing enteropathy and increased tissue demand are possible explanations (Sandford-Smith and Whittle 1979). Measles infection depresses cell mediated and humoral immunity, which may explain the secondary herpetic infection (Aaby *et al.* 1987). Traditional eye medicines can cause corneal ulceration from thermal and chemical burns, physical trauma, and by introducing secondary bacterial or fungal infection.

MEASLES IMMUNIZATION

In industrialized countries low-titre, live attenuated measles vaccines are safe, immunogenic and effective when given in the second year of life. The vaccines are made from the Edmonston strain of virus, and the Schwartz vaccine is the most commonly used. The currently available vaccines are heat and light labile and have to be stored at 4°C; a 'cold chain' is therefore required. In developing countries the usually recommended age for immunization is 9 months. Immunization is ineffective before the age of 4 months due to the presence of maternal antibodies. This leaves a window of high risk for infants aged between 4 and 9 months (Tidjani *et al.* 1989). Different vaccines (*e.g.* the Edmonston–Zagreb), different titres and timing schedules for measles immunization are currently being evaluated to determine the best regimen for countries where measles is a significant cause of death before the age of 9 months (Aaby *et al.* 1988, Tidjani *et al.* 1989, Whittle *et al.* 1990, Kiepiela *et al.* 1991).

Measles immunization programmes have been introduced in many developing countries as part of the WHO Extended Programme of Immunization. The aim is to achieve a minimum coverage of 80 per cent: this is currently being reached in some but not all countries. Barriers to successful immunization programmes include competing health priorities, poor primary health care infrastructure, low health worker motivation, difficulties in maintaining the cold chain, population migration, and low levels of education and awareness among parents.

PREVENTIVE STRATEGIES

(1) Primary prevention:
   —measles immunization;
   —health education regarding the use of traditional eye medicines.
(2) Secondary prevention (prevention of corneal scarring from measles infection):
   —high dose vitamin A treatment of all children with measles;
   —antibiotic treatment for secondary infection;
   —antiviral agents for HSV keratitis.
(3) Tertiary prevention (restoration of vision due to corneal scarring from measles):
   —optical iridectomy;
   —corneal grafting.

Ophthalmia neonatorum

Ophthalmia neonatorum (ON) was a major cause of childhood blindness in England and other European countries at the end of the last century (Jay 1987, Fransen and Klauss 1988). The introduction of silver nitrate prophylaxis (Credé's method) in 1884 was probably the prime factor responsible for the virtual elimination of this cause of childhood blindness at the turn of the century. Very few data on ON are available from developing countries, mainly because of difficulties in obtaining accurate details of medical histories.

The prevalence of gonorrhoea and genital chlamydial infection among women attending antenatal clinics in African countries ranges from 3 to 22 per cent and from 1 to 18 per cent respectively. Approximately 30 per cent and 25 to 50 per cent of infants exposed to *Neisseria gonorrhoeae* and *Chlamydia trachomatis* during birth develop gonococcal or chlamydial conjunctivitis. The incidence of gonococcal ON in European countries is approximatley 0.04 to 0.3 per 1000 live births, as compared with 40/1000 in Kenya and the Cameroon. The higher incidence in African countries reflects the higher incidence of sexually transmitted diseases, which are frequently undetected and untreated, and lack of ocular prophylaxis in the newborn (Fransen and Klauss 1988, Laga *et al.* 1989). Gonococcal ON tends to appear earlier and be more severe than chlamydial infection. In a clinic based study, 16 per cent of babies with gonococcal ON had corneal involvement (Laga *et al.* 1989).

TREATMENT OF SEXUALLY TRANSMITTED DISEASE DURING PREGNANCY

Treatment of gonorrhoea has been complicated by the emergence of penicillin resistant strains and strains resistant to tetracycline and some of the earlier cephalosporins (Haimovici and Roussel 1989). The incidence of penicillin resistant strains is low in industrialized countries but may be as high as 80 per cent in developing countries, particularly in Africa (Lepage *et al.* 1988). In areas where the prevalence of such strains is less than 1 per cent, infected pregnant women and their partners should receive full treatment with high dose intramuscular benzylpenicillin (4.8 million IU) with probenecid 1g orally, or systemic tetracycline, doxycycline or ampicillin. In areas where strains have reduced the efficacy of these antimicrobials to below 95 per cent, other antibiotics, such as third generation cephalosporins, are required (WHO 1986).

OCULAR PROPHYLAXIS AND TREATMENT OF OPHTHALMIA NEONATORUM

Ocular prophylaxis involves careful cleansing of the eylids as soon as the head is delivered and before the eyes open, followed by instillation of an antiseptic or antibiotic. No perfect medication exists for this purpose, but the main choices are 1% silver nitrate drops, and tetracycline and erythromycin ointment. Silver nitrate is active against all strains of *N. gonorrhoeae*, regardless of antibiotic sensitivity, is inexpensive, widely available and easy to apply. It is not effective against *C. trachomatis*, however, and causes chemical conjunctivitis in up to 90 per cent of

190

infants. Tetracycline ointment is as effective as silver nitrate in preventing gonococcal ON, and is also active against chlamydial ON. Tetracycline is widely available but some strains of *N. gonorrhoeae* are resistant (WHO 1986). Erythromycin ointment is effective at preventing gonococcal and chlamydial ON, but is not widely available (Lund *et al.* 1987).

Treatment of ON should be initiated immediately, without waiting for results of bacteriological investigations. Intensive topical and systemic treatment is required; treatment can be modified later after the responsible organism/s has/have been identified and drug sensitivity determined. In developing countries where the incidence of resistant strains is high, where antibiotics are not readily available and where compliance with treatment is likely to be poor, the ideal treatment would consist of a single systemic dose of antibiotic. Kanamycin combined with topical tetracycline has been recommended by WHO (1986) but its ototoxicity has not been sufficiently investigated. Recent evidence suggests that single-dose treatment with third generation cephalosporins, such as cefoxamine and ceftriaxone, may be equally effective and have fewer side-effects. They are effective without additional topical treatment and also clear extraocular foci of infection (Laga *et al.* 1986, Lepage *et al.* 1988).

In areas where the prevalence of infection caused by penicillin resistent *N. gonorrhoeae* strains is less than 1 per cent, WHO (1986) have recommended the following treatment schedule: topical penicillin drops or tetracycline ointment, combined with intramuscular benzylpenicillin 50,000 U/kg in two divided doses per day for two days. In areas of higher prevalence, the recommended schedule is kanamycin 25mg/kg combined with topical treatment, or a single intramuscular dose of cefotaxime 100mg/kg.

Conjunctivitis of the newborn is becoming an increasingly serious problem in developing countries for several reasons. Firstly, infected pregnant women are frequently not identified and treated; secondly, agents for ocular prophylaxis are often not available, have been discontinued, or are applied to only a small proportion of newborn babies because most deliveries take place outside hospitals or clinics; thirdly, an increasing number of strains of *N. gonorrhoeae* are resistant to penicillin and tetracycline; and lastly, antibiotic treatment for ON is not generally available, and if the infection is caused by a resistant strain, treatment will not be effective. To reduce the problem of blindness from ON, prophylactic agents and antibiotics which are safe, effective and cheap must be made available to all levels of health care, particularly to village health workers and traditional birth attenders for babies born at home.

PREVENTIVE STRATEGIES
(1) Primary prevention:
    —prevention of sexually transmitted diseases, by health education, etc.;
    —identification and antibiotic treatment of sexually transmitted diseases in pregnant women;

—cleansing of newborn babies' eyelids immediately after birth;
—ocular prophylaxis in the newborn, *e.g.* 1% silver nitrate solution, tetracycline ointment.
(2) Secondary prevention:
—early identification of ON, and appropriate treatment with topical and systemic antibiotics.
(3) Tertiary prevention:
—corneal graft;
—optical iridectomy.

Blindness from cataract

Blind school studies show that cataracts account for 3 to 39 per cent of childhood blindness (Foster 1988), with an estimated 200,000 children being blind from this cause (Table 16.5). In industrialized countries, stimulus deprivation amblyopia is the main cause of visual loss, due to delayed surgery, inaccurate aphakic correction and inadequate occlusion therapy (Taylor 1979, Taylor and Rice 1982). In developing countries, blindness also results from unoperated cataract and complications following surgery.

Blind school studies in West Africa and India show that 9 and 3 per cent respectively of the blind school populations had bilateral unoperated cataract (personal data, unpublished). The majority of aphakic children did not have corrective glasses.

Aetiology

In the UK approximately 50 per cent of childhood cataract is idiopathic, 20 per cent is due to genetic disease, and in the remaining 30 per cent cataracts are found in association with other ocular abnormalities, *e.g.* retinal dysplasia, persistent primary hyperplastic vitreous and retinal dystrophies, or in association with syndromes or chromosomal abnormalities, *e.g.* congenitally acquired rubella and Down syndrome (Hing *et al.* 1990). This is in contrast to the findings of a blind school study in Jamaica where 39 per cent of children were blind from cataract. In this population 48 per cent of cataract blindness was attributed to rubella and 33 per cent to hereditary factors (Moriarty 1988). In a blind school study in West Africa, 15 per cent of children were blind from cataract. Congenitally acquired rubella accounted for 15 per cent of cases, and in 16 per cent there was a positive family history (personal data, unpublished). Few data are available from other parts of the world on the aetiology of non-traumatic childhood cataract. There is evidence, however, that congenitally acquired rubella has become an unusual cause of congenital cataract in countries with rubella immunization programmes (Hing *et al.* 1990).

Management

The management of congenital cataract is complex, as surgery to clear the visual axis must be followed by prompt and accurate aphakic correction, and rigorous treatment and follow-up to prevent amblyopia (Taylor 1981). Good health care services and certain socioeconomic advantages are essential, which may not be available in developing countries.

The surgical management of congenital cataract has evolved as new and better techniques, such as extracapsular extraction and lensectomy, have been introduced (Taylor 1981, 1982, 1985; Keech *et al.* 1989). In developing countries the techniques of needling, linear extraction and aspiration are still frequently used. Each method has potential per- and postoperative complications. Needling and linear extraction are associated with a high incidence of postoperative uveitis and pupil block glaucoma (Chandler 1968), and secondary procedures may be required to remove residual soft lens matter and to clear the visual axis. Posterior capsular opacification occurs in the majority, requiring capsulotomy (Sheppard and Crawford 1973). Late complications, *i.e.* secondary glaucoma and retinal detachment, occur more often in eyes on which multiple operations have been performed (Phelps and Arafat 1977, Toyofuku *et al.* 1980). Lens aspiration and extracapsular extraction have fewer postoperative complications, but posterior capsule opacification frequently occurs. This prevents accurate refraction, delays aphakic correction and blurs the visual image (Parks 1984). Capsulotomy is required, either surgically or using a YAG laser. During lensectomy the majority of the lens and capsular bag are removed, and a limited anterior vitrectomy is usually performed (Peyman *et al.* 1978). Peroperative and early and late postoperative complications are fewer, and the optical axis is clear from the first postoperative day (Peyman *et al.* 1978, Douvas 1981, Nelson 1984), but whether the long term complications of glaucoma and retinal detachment are fewer remains to be seen.

The aims of surgery are to clear the visual axis to permit accurate refraction and optimal optical correction as stimulus deprivation amblyopia is minimal if the refractive error is corrected immediately after surgery. Options for aphakic correction include spectacles, contact lenses, intraocular lenses and epikeratophakia (Dutton *et al.* 1990). Aphakic refractive errors change rapidly during infancy and early childhood, necessitating frequent refraction and adjustment of the aphakic correction (Dutton *et al.* 1990). This is possible with contact lenses and spectacles, but not with intraocular lenses and epikeratophakia. Continuous-wear soft contact lenses give the best visual results, but intensive follow-up is required to change the prescription and to replace missing lenses. Good hygiene is required as infective corneal ulceration can occur which makes this option a potentially hazardous one in developing countries. Spectacles are cheap and easy to change and replace, but are difficult to fit on small babies. The role of intraocular lenses is controversial as the technique is difficult in children and the long-term complications are not known (Menezo *et al.* 1985, Dutton *et al.* 1990). Epikeratophakia is a new technique currently being used in children intolerant of contact lenses (Menezo *et al.* 1985).

Visual results following childhood cataract surgery have improved due to advances in surgical techniques and changes in management to prevent stimulus deprivation amblyopia. Better results are obtained in simple cataracts (*i.e.* where there are no associated ocular abnormalities), by early surgery using the techniques of extracapsular extraction and lensectomy, and by prompt aphakic correction (Peyman *et al.* 1981, Pratt-Johnson and Tillson 1981, Parks 1982, Taylor 1982, Hing *et al.* 1990). However, very little information concerning the outcome of childhood cataract surgery is available from developing countries, only two small studies having been published. One retrospective study from India reported findings in 70 children, of whom 53 had unilateral idiopathic or traumatic cataract and 17 had bilateral cataracts. No surgical details were reported, nor was the outcome analysed according to type of cataract, age at surgery or method of aphakic correction (Shrivastva *et al.* 1988). In the other study, also from India, 20 out of 50 children undergoing needling for bilateral cataracts had acuities of less than 6/60 at follow-up (Jain *et al.* 1983). Poor visual results were attributed to amblyopia, posterior capsule opacification and retinal detachment. The importance and difficulties of good follow-up and compliance in this setting were stressed.

Preliminary findings of a retrospective study of 103 children with congenital cataract in India show that only 41 per cent presented before the age of 12 months. 15 per cent did not return for follow-up, and a further 52 per cent only attended for one or two appointments (personal data, unpublished). This highlights the problems of preventing cataract blindness in children in developing countries.

Preventive strategies
(1) Primary prevention:
   —rubella immunization;
   —genetic counselling and family planning;
   —antenatal diagnosis of genetic disease and chromosomal abnormalities with termination of pregnancy.
(2) Secondary prevention:
   —early identification of neonates and infants with cataracts;
   —early surgery, prompt accurate aphakic correction, occlusion therapy.
(3) Tertiary prevention:
   —identification of older children with unoperated cataract;
   —late surgery to restore navigational vision;
   —appropriate optical aids to maximize use of residual vision.

Blindness from retinopathy of prematurity
ROP emerged as a cause of childhood blindness in the late 1940s and the 1950s, due to improvements in neonatal care and increased survival of preterm babies. During the 1950s ROP was the single most common cause of childhood blindness in many industrialized countries. Hyperoxia was proposed as an important aetiological factor (Campbell 1951) which was largely supported by laboratory research and clinical trials (Flynn 1987). The use of oxygen was restricted in the mid-50s, which

was followed by a reduction in the incidence of blindness from ROP, but a higher infant mortality rate (Cross 1973). Oxygen was used more liberally again in the 1960s, and blindness from ROP began to re-emerge. The introduction of increasingly sophisticated technology and accurate methods of monitoring blood oxygen levels in the 1970s were probably the major factors responsible for the reduction in blinding ROP observed during this period.

The risk of ROP is inversely related to gestational age and birthweight. More very low birthweight (VLBW, <1500g) and extremely low birthweight (ELBW, <1000g) babies are being born, and their survival rates continue to improve due to advances in neonatal care (Patz 1983). The population of babies at risk for ROP is therefore increasing. There is recent evidence to suggest that blindness from ROP is also increasing in some countries.

Two longitudinal, population based studies undertaken in Canada and Denmark provide evidence of an increasing incidence in blindness from ROP (Fledelius and Rosenberg 1990, Gibson et al. 1990). In the USA a 'second epidemic' of blindness from ROP is thought to be occurring (Phelps 1979). In the UK, however, information which might allow assessment of changing patterns of blindness from ROP is lacking, as accurate incidence data are not available. Data from community and hospital based studies show that the pattern of advanced ROP is changing, with more immature infants becoming blind (Linfield and Davies 1987, Schulenberg et al. 1987, Ben Sira et al. 1988, Ng et al. 1988, Seiberth and Linderkamp 1989, Stannard et al. 1989, Fledelius and Rosenberg 1990).

There is some evidence that ROP may be emerging in parts of Latin America, such as Chile (Gilbert et al. 1993a), and in urban areas of some of the newly industrialized countries of South-east Asia, such as Thailand and the Philippines (Gilbert and Foster 1993).

Pathogenesis and natural history
Case control studies have shown that the two major risk factors for ROP are preterm birth and hyperoxia (Ben Sira et al. 1988, Seiberth and Linderkamp 1989). Other associated factors include hypoxia, acidosis, intraventricular haemorrhage, vitamin E deficiency and septicaemia, although their pathogenic significance is unclear. Progression to advanced, blinding disease seems to be determined by the degree of immaturity of the retina and the severity of the early insult (Prendiville and Schulenberg 1988). A recent study of surfactant treatment for babies with respiratory distress syndrome (RDS) has shown a lower incidence of ROP in these babies than in a matched group without RDS (Rankin et al. 1992). Surfactant replacement therapy may have an important part to play in stabilizing the infant's homeostasis during the early critical period of life. Systemic steroids given in the period immediately before preterm birth can, under some circumstances, reduce the incidence of RDS (Liggins 1989), which may in turn lead to a reduction in the incidence of ROP.

In 1984 a classification system for ROP was introduced (Table 16.11), which

195

TABLE 16.11

Classification of retinopathy of prematurity by stage and extent*

Stage I	Demarcation line
Stage II	Ridge
Stage III	Ridge with extraretinal fibrovascular proliferation
Stage IV	Subtotal retinal detachment
	—a: extrafoveal detachment
	—b: foveal detachment
Stage V	Total retinal detachment
	—Anterior or posterior funnel
	—Open or closed funnel
Zone 1	Posterior pole
Zone 2	Retina extending peripherally to point tangential to nasal ora serrata
Zone 3	Temporal retinal periphery
'Plus' disease	Vascular incompetence
	Vitreous haze

*Committee for the Classification of ROP (1984).

takes into account both the severity of the disease (stages I–V), and the extent of changes (zones 1–3). An additional classification, 'plus' disease, is used to denote the presence of vascular incompetence and vitreous involvement (Committee for Classification of ROP 1984, Patz 1987).

Natural history studies show that the earliest signs of ROP begin six to eight weeks after birth; the disease process evolves over the next two to five weeks (Schulenberg *et al.* 1987), with spontaneous regression commonly occurring in stages I, II and early stage III. Blindness results from progression to stage IV or stage V disease, or from cicatricial consequences of regressed disease (Patz 1987). Disease in zone 1 carries a worse prognosis than disease in zones 2 or 3. An important sign which indicates that stage III may progress to stage IV or V is the development of 'plus' disease. Once the vitreous becomes involved, retinal detachment develops within two to three weeks in 50 per cent of cases. Hospital based studies have shown that the proportion of low birthweight preterm babies with ROP of all stages can reach 60 per cent (Linfield and Davies 1987), rising to 72 per cent in ELBW babies (Charles *et al.* 1991). The proportion of VLBW babies with Stage III 'plus' disease and subsequent blindness can be as high as 11 per cent (Acheson and Schulenberg 1991) and 8 per cent (Fledelius 1990) respectively. Selection bias due to different referral patterns, standards of neonatal care and selection criteria for neonatal intensive care, as well as observer bias, may account for the variation in reported incidence.

Treatment

Recent clinical trials have shown that peripheral retinal cryotherapy for babies with

196

threshold disease (*i.e.* five or more contiguous clock hours or eight or more non-contiguous clock hours of stage III 'plus' disease) can prevent progression to blinding disease. The American Multicenter Trial, which randomly allocated babies with stage III 'plus' disease to receive cryotherapy or no treatment, showed that treatment had a favourable outcome in 46 per cent of cases (Cryotherapy for ROP Cooperative Group 1990). Other, uncontrolled trials suggest that earlier intervention, before 'plus' disease develops, may be of benefit (Nissenkorn *et al.* 1991). Laser photocoagulation is also effective and probably less traumatic than cryotherapy (Iverson *et al.* 1990). The outcome of complex vitreoretinal surgery for stages IV and V disease has recently been reviewed, indicating very disappointing functional results, even if the operation resulted in retinal reattachment (Kalina 1991).

With the introduction of an effective and safe treatment it is important to identify babies at risk of blindness, *i.e.* those with stage III 'plus' disease, so that treatment can be given. A Working Group of the College of Ophthalmologists, London, has proposed guidelines for screening, recommending which babies should be examined and the timing of examinations (Levene *et al.* 1990). In the UK, an estimated 450 babies per year are at risk of blindness (Levene *et al.* 1990), and without treatment 50 to 100 babies will become bilaterally blind each year.

Preventive strategies
(1) Primary prevention:
    —good antenatal care to prevent preterm birth;
    —good neonatal care;
    —?surfactant replacement therapy.
(2) Secondary prevention:
    —screening to identify babies with treatable disease;
    —cryotherapy/laser photocoagulation.
(3) Tertiary prevention:
    —complex vitreoretinal surgery (usually unsuccessful in restoring sight).
Some of the potential barriers to preventing blindness from ROP are the levels of staff, training, time and equipment necessary to provide good neonatal care and for screening, monitoring and treating affected babies. These factors pose particular problems for moderately developed countries where there may be other health priorities, and limited personnel and financial resources.

Blindness from genetic disease
In industrialized countries genetic disease and chromosomal abnormalities account for approximately half of all cases of childhood blindness, the principal conditions being tapetoretinal degenerations, macular dystrophies, cataracts, optic atrophy and albinism (Halldorsson and Bjornsson 1980, Kavanozi and Tsikoulas 1986, Van der Pol 1986, Jay 1987, Phillips *et al.* 1987, Rosenberg 1987, Goggin and O'Keefe 1991, Rosenberg *et al.* 1992). Genetic disease assumes greater importance now than

earlier in the century mainly because of a reduction in blindness from conditions that are more readily preventable or treatable, such as ophthalmia neonatorum and cataract. The limited data available from developing countries (see Table 16.4) suggest that genetic factors are responsible for a lower proportion of childhood blindness than in the industrialized nations. This probably reflects the higher prevalence of acquired causes of blindness rather than a lower incidence of genetic disease, but epidemiological data to support this are not available.

Marriage between close relatives is practised in many parts of the world, with up to 50 per cent of marriages being consanguineous in some societies. The 'inbreeding coefficient' indicates the proportion of autosomal loci predicted from pedigree analysis to be homozygous through inheritance of identical genes from a common ancestor. For example, the offspring of a first-cousin marriage are likely to be homozygous at approximately 6 per cent (*i.e.* 1/16 or $1/2^4$) of gene loci. The consequence of consanguineous marriage is a higher incidence of autosomal recessive disease. If the homozygous state is deleterious this may adversely influence the individual's capacity for survival and reproduction (fitness). If the gene is not deleterious when heterozygous, it will not be 'bred out' by selection if new mutations occur at the same rate to compensate for loss of deleterious alleles (the mutational model). Conversely, the heterozygote state may confer increased fitness, maintaining the gene in the population, *e.g.* the sickle cell trait confers protection against malaria (the segregational model). The pattern of genetic disease found in a population depends on the size and degree of isolation of the population, the nature of the genetic abnormalities present in the gene pool, and the extent of consanguineous marriage. For example, Tay–Sachs disease is found almost exclusively amongst Ashkenazi Jews.

Genetic abnormalities can be inherited as autosomal dominant or recessive traits, or be X-linked, or be inherited through abnormalities in mitochondrial DNA. An example of the latter is Leber's optic neuropathy. The type of inheritance can usually be determined by pedigree studies, which should include clinical examination and/or biochemical testing, to identify carriers and those with mild disease. Sporadic cases of disease can occur, due to rare autosomal recessive or X-linked disease, or to a new mutation. Sporadic cases may not have a genetic basis but may mimic typical genetic disease (a phenocopy). Some conditions are genetically influenced, but are not inherited according to simple mendelian genetics. Disease may result from the additive effect of many different genes with or without the influence of environmental factors (multifactorial and polygenic inheritance respectively) (Gelehrter and Collins 1990). In a recent blind school study in Scotland, 42, 7 and 5 per cent of children were blind from autosomal dominant, recessive and X-linked disease respectively (Phillips *et al.* 1987).

Some genetic disease manifests itself at birth, *e.g.* trisomy 21 (Down syndrome) and malformations or structural abnormalities of the eye such as microphthalmos with coloboma and oculocutaneous albinism. Other diseases become manifest only later in life, *e.g.* dominant forms of retinitis pigmentosa.

Molecular basis

Knowledge and understanding of the molecular basis of genetic disease have increased rapidly over the last few years, and techniques have been developed which allow accurate localization and sequencing of genes and identification and localization of chromosomal and DNA abnormalities. Detailed descriptions of these techniques are beyond the scope of this review, but they include chromosomal karyotype analysis, and the use of restriction enzymes and recombinant DNA techniques for gene mapping. Southern blotting of cDNA derived from RNA can be used to create gene libraries, which may be tissue specific. Genetic abnormalities can be identified using the technique of restriction fragment length polymorphism (RFLP), and localized by linkage studies, using radioactively labelled probes (Wong 1987). Another method used to identify genetic abnormalities is the candidate gene approach: genes are selected which are specifically expressed in diseased tissue, or that are known to code for proteins with an important function in that tissue, and patients with the disease are then screened for mutations in each of these genes (Dryja 1992). The polymerase chain reaction technique amplifies chosen sequences of DNA so that genetic studies can be undertaken on very small samples such as might be obtained from venous blood samples, buccal mucosal scrapes, chorionic villus biopsy and cells obtained by amniocentesis.

The sites of abnormality have been localized for a number of ocular diseases (Musarella 1992), *e.g.* retinoblastoma, to band 14 of the long arm of chromosome 13 (13q14); aniridia, to band 13 of the short arm of chormosome 11 (11p13); and colour blindness, to band 28 of the long arm of the X chromosome (Xq28). Over 30 different mutations in the rhodopsin gene (on the long arm of chromosome 3) have been identified in families with autosomal dominant retinitis pigmentosa (Dryja 1992). However, only 25 to 30 per cent of families studied to date carry a mutation in the rhodopsin gene; the nature and site of abnormality in the other families is still to be determined. Autosomal dominant retinitis pigmentosa clearly demonstrates that a particular phenotype may be due to many different genetic abnormalities. Knowledge of the molecular basis of genetic disease is important not only because it can improve understanding of disease mechanisms and allow a rational approach to therapy, but also because the information can be used for disease prevention, by genetic counselling.

Prevention

A detailed family history, combined with examination of relevant family members and investigation where necessary, to determine the mode of inheritance and calculate risks in subsequent pregnancies are essential early steps in genetic counselling.

The techniques outlined above can then be used to provide presymptomatic diagnosis, and to identify carriers of X-linked and autosomal recessive traits. Appropriate genetic counselling gives prospective parents the option of limiting family size (primary prevention), or of starting a family with the knowledge that prenatal diagnosis may be a possibility, with termination of an affected pregnancy (secondary prevention). Prenatal diagnostic tests can be performed on samples obtained by chorionic villus biopsy during the first trimester of pregnancy, and by amniocentesis after 16 weeks.

The rapid advances that have been made in medical genetics mean that an increasing number of diseases with a genetic basis have the potential to be prevented. *In vitro* fertilization and preimplantation diagnosis, and somatic cell line therapy and even germ line therapy are possibilities for the future. However, many of the issues surrounding genetic counselling provoke complex moral, ethical and emotional problems. The main purpose of genetic counselling is to provide as much information as possible to families with genetic disease so that they can make informed decisions, and to provide support to those who are confronted with these difficult decisions.

PREVENTIVE STRATEGIES
(1) Primary prevention:
    —prevent pregnancy in families with autosomal dominant conditions, and in X-linked and recessive disease, after identification of carriers
    —(preimplantation diagnosis)
    —(germ line therapy)
(2) Secondary prevention:
    —prenatal diagnosis and termination of pregnancy;
    —early identification and treatment of genetic disease, *e.g.* congenital cataract;
    —(somatic cell line therapy).
(3) Tertiary prevention:
    —appropriate treatment, *e.g.* cataract surgery.

Blindness from cerebral and optic nerve disease

Recent data on causes of blindness in newly registered children in the UK shows that 52 of 235 children (22 per cent) were blind from disorders of the higher visual pathways, and a further 48 (20 per cent) from optic atrophy (Department of Health 1991). The aetiology of the cerebral and optic nerve disease was not stated. Studies in European countries report 15 to 54 per cent of children to be blind from central nervous system (CNS) abnormalities (Halldorsson and Bjornsson 1980, Kavanozi and Tsikoulas 1986, Van der Pol 1986, Phillips *et al.* 1987, Rosenberg 1987, Goggin and O'Keefe 1992). The high figure of 54 per cent was reported from a study of blind children in Eire, where the population comprised not only children registered as blind but also unregistered children (60 per cent of total) from institutions for the mutiply disabled (Goggin and O'Keefe 1991).

Data from developing countries show a much lower proportion of children to be blind from CNS disease, which may reflect either a lower incidence, or a high mortality rate, or be due to the higher prevalence of blindness from other causes.

Visual loss from CNS disease in developing countries has been attributed principally to optic atrophy (Foster 1988), but cerebral lesions without optic atrophy will undoubtedly have been missed in some children, since diagnoses were made clinically.

Aetiology

In the European studies listed above, the diagnoses included metabolic and genetic disease, intrauterine factors such as the toxic effects of alcohol, intrapartum events associated with birth asphyxia, and postnatal factors, including trauma, tumours and meningitis. Up to 59 per cent of children blind from CNS disease had additional impairments, most commonly cerebral palsy (CP) (Halldorsson and Bjornsson 1980, Rosenberg 1987, Goggin and O'Keefe 1991). Conversely CNS lesions were the most common cause (30 per cent) of blindness in 156 visually and mentally impaired children in the Netherlands (Copper and Schuppert-Kimmijser 1970).

Hypoxia resulting from intrapartum events has frequently been recorded as the underlying cause of both blindness and CP. However, there is now a body of evidence which indicates that clinical indicators of birth asphyxia, such as a low Apgar score and low umbilical pH, are very poor predictors of neurological abnormality (Paneth 1986, *Lancet* 1989). In one study in Australia only 8 per cent of cases of CP were attributed to intrapartum events (Blair and Stanley 1988). Longitudinal population based studies have also shown that the incidence of CP in babies with normal birthweight has not declined despite significant improvements in obstetric care. The underlying cause of CP in many children with normal birthweight seems to be related to ill-defined events or processes occurring before birth which either cause prenatal cerebral damage, or which make the cerebrum susceptible to damage from stresses during delivery. These observations have implications for understanding the origins of blindness in this group of children.

In developing countries it is often difficult to ascertain the underlying cause of blinding CNS abnormalities, but where the diagnosis is known the majority of cases appear to be due to postnatal events, *e.g.* meningitis (personal data, unpublished).

Preterm birth

The incidence of cerebral damage with CP and visual loss is higher in babies with low birthweight and in those born at or before 32 weeks gestation (Burgess and Johnson 1991, Escobar *et al.* 1991, Veen *et al.* 1991). Periventricular ischaemia and paraventricular and intraventricular haemorrhage are found in a high percentage of preterm babies, particularly those weighing <1000g at birth (Fujiwara *et al.* 1990). Severe lesions are associated with a high risk of subsequent disability and visual loss, which raises the difficult ethical question as to whether in some circumstances 'good neonatal care' may imply selective care. Once again there is debate concerning the aetiological significance and interrelationship of prenatal, intra-partum and neonatal events (Singha *et al.* 1990). Preterm birth may itself be a

TABLE 16.12
Summary of strategies for the control of childhood blindness

Disorder	Primary prevention	Secondary prevention	Tertiary prevention
Corneal scarring	Breast feeding Nutrition education Measles immunization Vit. A prophylaxis	High dose vit. A	Optical iridectomy (corneal graft)
Ophthalmia neonatorum	Health education Antenatal care Prophylaxis in newborn	Topical/systemic antibiotics	(Corneal graft)
Cataract	Rubella immunization Genetic counselling	Early surgery and optical correction	Late surgery and optical correction
Glaucoma	Rubella immunization	Early surgery	—
ROP	Good antenatal and neonatal care ?Surfactants	Cryotherapy Laser	—

reflection of adverse prenatal events as well as predisposing the immature infant to damage caused by haemodynamic, respiratory and metabolic stresses during birth and the neonatal period. There is some evidence that despite increased survival rates among VLBW babies, this does not seem to be associated with an increased incidence of disability (Grogaard *et al.* 1990), suggesting that at least some of the sequelae of preterm birth may be attributable to neonatal events which can, in part, be prevented by advanced neonatal care.

There is also a higher incidence of other causes of visual loss in children born preterm, including refractive errors, amblyopia and optic nerve hypoplasia (Hungerford *et al.* 1986, Burgess and Johnson 1991).

Preventive strategies
(1) Primary prevention:
  —good obstetric care to prevent avoidable causes of prenatal cerebral damage and preterm birth;
  —good intensive neonatal care;
  —genetic counselling to prevent inherited disease.
(2) Secondary prevention:
  —appropriate treatment of hydrocephalus, meningitis, encephalitis, intracranial neoplasms, etc.

Summary
Many of the causes of childhood blindness are avoidable, *i.e.* are amenable to primary and secondary preventive measures. This is particularly true of developing countries where up to 70 per cent of childhood blindness is avoidable (Foster and

Gilbert 1992, Gilbert *et al.* 1993*a*). Strategies for primary, secondary and tertiary prevention to reduce childhood blindness from various causes are summarized in Table 16.12. In developing countries the relevant primary preventive strategies, such as nutrition education, vitamin A supplementation and measles immunization can be provided through child survival programmes. In industrialized countries, strategies for prevention require close cooperation and communication between the health care professionals who look after babies and young children, including obstetricians, neonatologists, paediatricians, ophthalmologists and medical geneticists. Secondary preventive measures require the early identification of neonates and children with treatable conditions and referral to centres which can provide the appropriate ophthalmic care. Tertiary prevention is more problematic in children with early onset disease because of amblyopia. Useful vision can usually be restored to a child blind from unoperated congenital cataract, and occasionally optical iridectomy or keratoplasty can restore sight to a child blind from corneal scarring.

REFERENCES

Aaby, P. (1988) *Malnourished or Overinfected. An Analysis of the Determinants of Acute Measles Mortality.* Copenhagen: Lægeforeningens Forlag.
—— Bukh, J., Hoff, G., Lisse, I.M., Smits, A.J. (1987) 'Humoral immunity in measles infection: a critical factor?' *Medical Hypotheses*, **23**, 287–310.
—— Hansen, H.L., Sodemann, M., Knudsen, K.M., Jensen, T.G., Kristiansen, H., Poulsen, A., Jakobsen, M., da Silva, M.C., Whittle, H.C. (1988) 'Trial of high-dose Edmonston-Zagreb measles vaccine in Guinea-Bissau: protective efficacy.' *Lancet*, **2**, 809-814.
Acheson, J.F., Schulenberg, W.E. (1991) 'Surveillance for retinopathy of prematurity in practice: experience from one neonatal intensive care unit.' *Eye*, **5**, 80–85.
Animashaun, A. (1977) 'Measles blindness in Nigerian children.' *Nigerian Journal of Paediatrics*, **4**, 10–13.
Ben Sira, I., Nissenkorn, I., Kremer, I. (1988) 'Retinopathy of prematurity.' *Survey of Ophthalmology*, **33**, 1–16.
Blair, E., Stanley, F.J. (1988) 'Intrapartum asphyxia: a rare cause of cerebral palsy.' *Journal of Pediatrics*, **112**, 515–519.
Brilliant, G.E. (Ed.) (1988) *The Epidemiology of Blindness in Nepal. Report of the 1981 Nepal Blindness Survey.* Chelsea, MI: Seva Foundation.
Burgess, P., Johnson, A. (1991) 'Ocular defects in infants of extremely low birth weight and gestational age.' *British Journal of Ophthalmology*, **75**, 84–87.
Campbell, K. (1951) 'Intensive oxygen therapy as a possible cause of retrolental fibroplasia: a clinical approach.' *Medical Journal of Australia*, **2**, 48–50.
Chandler, P.A. (1968) 'Surgery of congenital cataract. The 24th Jackson Memorial Lecture.' *American Journal of Ophthalmology*, **65**, 663–674.
Charles, J.B., Ganthier, R., Appiah, A.P. (1991) 'Incidence and characteristics of retinopathy of prematurity in a low-income inner-city population.' *Ophthalmology*, **98**, 14–17.
Chirambo, M.C., Tielsch, J.M., West, K.P., Katz, J., Tizazu, T., Schwab, L., Johnson, G., Swartwood, J., Taylor, H.R., Sommer A. (1986) 'Blindness and visual impairment in southern Malawi.' *Bulletin of the World Health Organization*, **64**, 567–572.
Cohen, N., Rahman, H., Sprague, J., Jahl, M., Leambujis, E., Mitra, M. (1985) 'Prevalence and determinants of nutritional blindness in Bangladeshi children.' *World Health Statistics Quarterly*, **38**, 317–329.
Committee for the Classification of Retinopathy of Prematurity (1984) 'An international classification system of retinopathy of prematurity.' *Archives of Ophthalmology*, **102**, 1130–1134.

Copper, A.C., Schuppert-Kimmijser, J. (1970) 'The causes of blindness in 156 visually and mentally defective children.' *Ophthalmologica*, **160**, 292–302.

Cross, K.W. (1973) 'Cost of preventing retrolental fibroplasia.' *Lancet*, **2**, 954–956.

Cryotherapy for Retinopathy of Prematurity Cooperative Group (1990) 'Multicenter trial of cryotherapy for retinopathy of prematurity. One year outcome—structure and function.' *Archives of Ophthalmology*, **108**, 1408–1416.

Daulaire, N.M.P., Starbuck, E.S., Houston, R.M., Church, M.S., Stukel, T.A. (1992) 'Childhood mortality after a high dose of vitamin A in a high risk population.' *British Medical Journal*, **304**, 207–210.

Department of Health (1991) *Causes of Blindness and Partial Sight Among Children Aged Under 16, Newly Registered as Blind and Partially Sighted Between April 1987 and March 1990.* Stanmore, Middlesex: Department of Health Information Division. (Statistical bulletin 3.5.91.)

Douvas, N.G. (1981) 'Phakectomy with shallow anterior vitrectomy in congenital and juvenile cataracts.' *Developments in Ophthalmology*, **2**, 163–174.

Dryja, T.P. (1992) 'Doyne Lecture. Rhodopsin and autosomal dominant retinitis pigmentosa.' *Eye*, **6**, 1–10.

Dutton, J.J., Baker, J.D., Hiles, D.A., Morgan, K.S. (1990) 'Visual rehabilitation in aphakic children.' *Survey of Ophthalmology*, **34**, 365–384.

Escobar, G.J., Littenberg, B., Petitti, D.B. (1991) 'Outcome among surviving very low birthweight infants: a meta-analysis.' *Archives of Disease in Childhood*, **66**, 204–211.

Faal, H., Minassian, D., Sowa, S., Foster, A. (1989) 'National survey of blindness and low vision in The Gambia.' *British Journal of Ophthalmology*, **73**, 82–87.

Fairney, A., Sloan, M.A., Patel, K.V., Coumbe, A. (1987) 'Vitamin A and D status of black South African women and their babies.' *Human Nutrition—Clinical Nutrition*, **41**, 81–87.

Fledelius, H.C. (1990) 'Retinopathy of prematurity. Clinical findings in a Danish county 1982–87.' *Acta Ophthalmologica*, **68**, 209–213.

—— Rosenberg, T. (1990) 'Retinopathy of prematurity. Where to set the screening limits? Recommendations based on two Danish surveys.' *Acta Paediatrica Scandinavia*, **79**, 906–910.

Flynn, J.T. (1987) 'Retinopathy of prematurity.' *Pediatric Clinics of North America*, **34**, 1487–1516.

Foster, A. (1988) 'Childhood blindness.' *Eye*, **2** (Suppl.), S27–S36.

—— Gilbert, C. (1992) 'Epidemiology of childhood blindness.' *Eye*, **6**, 173–176.

—— Sommer, A. (1986) 'Corneal ulceration, measles, and childhood blindness in Tanzania.' *British Journal of Ophthalmology*, **71**, 331–343.

Fransen, L., Klauss, V. (1988) 'Neonatal ophthalmia in the developing world.' *International Ophthalmology*, **11**, 189–196.

Fujiwara, T., Konishi, M., Chida, S., Okuyama, K., Ogawa, Y., Takeuchi, Y., Nishida, H., Kito, H., Fujimura, M., Nakamura, H., *et al.* (1990) 'Surfactant replacement therapy with a single postventilatory dose of a reconstituted bovine surfactant in preterm neonates with respiratory distress syndrome: final analysis of a multicenter, double-blind, randomized trial and comparison with similar trials.' *Paediatrics*, **86**, 753–764.

Gadomski, A.M., Kjolhede, C.L., Wittpenn, J., Bulux, J., Roasa, A.R., Forman, M.R. (1989) 'Conjunctival impression cytology (CIC) to detect subclinical vitamin A deficiency: comparison of CIC with biochemical assessments.' *American Journal of Clinical Nutrition*, **49**, 495–500.

Garenne, M., Leroy, O., Beau, J-P., Sene, I. (1991) 'Child mortality after high titre measles vaccines: prospective study in Senegal.' *Lancet*, **338**, 903–920.

Gelehrter, T.D., Collins, F. (1990) 'The role of genetics in medicine.' *In:* Garder, J. (Ed.) *Principles of Medical Genetics*. Baltimore: Williams & Wilkins, pp. 1–7.

Gibson, D.L., Sheps, S.B., Uh, S.H., Schechter, M.T., McCormick, A.Q. (1990) 'Retinopathy of prematurity-induced blindness: birth weight-specific survival and the new epidemic.' *Pediatrics*, **86**, 405–412.

Gilbert, C., Foster, A. (1993) 'Causes of blindness in children attending four schools for the blind in Thailand and the Philippines: a comparison between urban and rural blind school populations.' *International Ophthalmology. (In press.)*

—— Canovas, R., Hagan, M., Rao, S., Foster, A. (1993*a*) 'Causes of childhood blindness: results from West Africa, South India and Chile.' *Eye*, **7**, 184–188.

—— Foster, A., Thylefors, B., Negrel, A.D. (1993*b*) 'Childhood blindness: a new form for recording causes of visual loss in children.' *Bulletin of the World Health Organization. (In press.)*

Goggin, M., O'Keefe, M. (1991) 'Childhood blindness in the Republic of Ireland: a national survey.' *British Journal of Ophthalmology*, **75**, 425–429.

Grogaard, J.B., Linstrom, D.P., Culley, B., Stahlman, J. (1990) 'Increased survival rate in very low birth weight infants (1,500 grams or less): no association with increased incidence of handicaps.' *Pediatrics*, **117**, 139–146.

Haimovici, R., Roussel, T.J. (1989) 'Treatment of gonococcal conjunctivitis with single dose intramuscular ceftriaxone.' *American Journal of Ophthalmology*, **107**, 511–514.

Halldorsson, S., Bjornsson, G. (1980) 'Childhood blindness in Iceland.' *Acta Ophthalmologica*, **58**, 237–242.

Henderson, R.H., Keja, J., Hayden, G., Galaazka, A., Clements, J., Chan, C. (1988) 'Immunizing the children of the world: progress and prospects.' *Bulletin of the World Health Organization*, **66**, 535–543.

Hing, S., Speedwell, L., Taylor, D. (1990) 'Lens surgery in infancy and childhood.' *British Journal of Ophthalmology*, **74**, 73–77.

Hungerford, J., Stewart, A., Hope, P. (1986) 'Ocular sequelae of preterm birth and their relationship to ultrasound evidence of cerebral damage.' *British Journal of Ophthalmology*, **70**, 463–468.

Iverson, D.A., Trese, M.T., Orgel, I.K., Williams, G.A., Oak, R. (1990) 'Laser photocoagulation for threshold retinopathy of prematurity.' *American Journal of Ophthalmology*, **110**, 429–431.

Jain, I.S., Pillai, P., Gangwar, D.N., Gopal, L., Dhir, S.P. (1983) 'Congenital cataract: management and results.' *Journal of Paediatric Ophthalmology and Strabismus*, **20**, 243–246.

Jay, B. (1987) 'Causes of blindness in school children.' *British Medical Journal*, **294**, 1183–1184.

Kalina, R.E. (1991) 'Treatment of retinal detachment due to retinopathy of prematurity. Documented disappointment.' *Ophthalmology*, **98**, 3–4.

Kavanozi, A., Tsikoulas, I. (1985) 'The changing aetiology of visual impairment in early childhood in Greece.' In: Jay, B. (Ed.) *Detection and Measurement of Visual Impairment in Pre-verbal Children. Documenta Ophthalmologica, Proceedings Series Vol. 45.* Dordrecht: Martinus Nijhoff, pp. 51–62.

Keech, R.V., Tongue, A.C., Scott, W.E. (1989) 'Complications after surgery for congenital and infantile cataracts.' *American Journal of Ophthalmology*, **108**, 136–141.

Kiepiela, P., Coovadia, H.M., Loemning, W.E.K., Coward, P., Botha, G., Hugo, J., Becker, P.J. (1991) 'Lack of efficacy of the standard potency Edmonston-Zagreb attenuated measles vaccine in African infants.' *Bulletin of the World Health Organization*, **69**, 221–227.

Kimati, V.P., Lyaruu, B. (1976) 'Measles complications as seen at Mwanza Regional Consultant and Teaching Hospital in 1973.' *East African Medical Journal*, **53**, 332–340.

Laga, M., Naamara, W., Brunham, R.C., D'Costa, L.J., Nsanze, H., Piot, P., Kunimoto, D., Ndinya-Achola, J.O., Slaney, L., Ronald, A.R., *et al.* (1986) 'Single-dose therapy of gonococcal ophthalmia neonatorum with ceftriaxone.' *New England Journal of Medicine*, **27**, 1382–1385.

—— Meheus, A., Piot, P. (1989) 'Epidemiology and control of gonococcal ophthalmia neonatorum.' *Bulletin of the World Health Organization*, **67**, 471–477.

Lancet (1989) 'Cerebral palsy, intrapartum care, and a shot in the foot.' *Lancet*, **2**, 1251–1252. *(Editorial.)*

Lepage, P., Bogaerts, J., Kestelyn, P. (1988) 'Single-dose cefotaxime intramuscularly cures gonococcal ophthalmia neonatorum.' *British Journal of Ophthalmology*, **72**, 518–520.

Levene, M., Garner, A., Johnston, S., Rennie, J., Schulenberg, E., Fielder, A. (1990) *Screening for Retinopathy of Prematurity.* Working Party Report, College of Ophthalmologists, London.

Liggins, G.C. (1989) 'Can the benefits of antepartum corticosteroid treatment be improved?' *European Journal of Obstetrics, Gynecology, and Reproductive Biology*, **33**, 25–30.

Linfield, P.B., Davies, J.G. (1987) 'Screening for retinopathy of prematurity.' *Ophthalmic Physiology and Optics*, **7**, 401–402.

Lund, R.J., Kibel, M.A., Knight, G.J., Van der Elst, C. (1987) Prophylaxis against gonococcal ophthalmia neonatorum. A prospective study.' *South African Medical Journal*, **72**, 620–621.

Menezo, J.L., Taboada, J.F., Ferrer, E. (1985) 'Complications of intraocular lenses in children.' *Transactions of the Ophthalmological Society of the United Kingdom*, **104**, 546–552.

Moriarty, B.J. (1988) 'Childhood blindness in Jamaica.' *British Journal of Ophthalmology*, **72**, 65–67.

Morley, D.C., Martin, W.J., Allen, I. (1967) 'Measles in East and Central Africa.' *East African Medical Journal*, **44**, 497–508.

205

Musarella, M. (1992) 'Gene mapping of ocular diseases.' *Survey of Ophthalmology*, **36**, 285–311.

Nelson, L.B. (1984) 'Diagnosis and management of cataracts in infancy and childhood.' *Ophthalmic Surgery*, **15**, 688–697.

Nelson, M. (1990) 'Vitamin A, liver consumption, and risk of birth defects.' *British Medical Journal*, **301**, 1176. (*Editorial*.)

Ng, Y.K., Shaw, D., Levene, M.I., Fielder, A.R. (1988) 'Epidemiology of retinopathy of prematurity.' *Lancet*, **2**, 1235–1238.

Nissenkorn, I., Axer-Siegel, R., Kremer, I., Ben-Sira, I. (1991) 'Effect of partial cryoablation on retinopathy of prematurity.' *British Journal of Ophthalmology*, **75**, 160–162.

Paneth, N. (1986) 'Birth and the origins of cerebral palsy.' *New England Journal of Medicine*, **315**, 124–126.

Parks, M.M. (1982) 'Visual results in aphakic children.' *American Journal of Ophthalmology*, **4**, 441–449.

—— (1984) 'Management of the posterior capsule in congenital cataracts.' *Journal of Pediatric Ophthalmology and Strabismus*, **21**, 114–116.

Patz, A. (1983) 'Current therapy of retrolental fibroplasia.' *Ophthalmology*, **90**, 425–427.

—— (1987) 'An international classification of retinopathy of prematurity. II: The classification of retinal detachment.' *Archives of Ophthalmology*, **105**, 905–912.

Pepping, F., Hackenitz, E.A., Mroso, D.M., Franken, S., West, C.E. (1987) 'The role of nutritional status with special reference to vitamin A in the development of post-measles eye lesions.' *In:* Pepping, F. *Xerophthalmia and Post-measles Eye Lesions in Children in Tanzania. A Study of Nutritional, Biochemical and Ophthalmological Aspects.* (Thesis, Landbouwuniversiteit te Wageningen, pp. 117–131.)

Peyman, G.A., Raichand, M., Goldberg, M.F. (1978) 'Surgery of congenital and juvenile cataracts: a pars plicata approach with the vitrophage.' *British Journal of Ophthalmology*, **62**, 780–783.

—— —— Oesterle, C., Goldberg, M.F. (1981) 'Pars plicata lensectomy and vitrectomy in the management of congenital cataracts.' *Ophthalmology*, **88**, 437–439.

Phelps, C.D., Arafat, N.I. (1977) 'Open-angle glaucoma following surgery for congenital cataracts.' *Archives of Ophthalmology*, **95**, 1985–1987.

Phelps, D.L. (1979) 'Retinopathy of prematurity: an estimate of vision loss in the United States.' *Pediatrics*, **67**, 924–926.

Phillips, C., Levy, A.M., Newton, M., Stokoe, N.L. (1987) 'Blindness in school children: importance of hereditary, congenital cataract and prematurity.' *British Journal of Ophthalmology*, **71**, 578–584.

Pratt-Johnson, J.A., Tillson, G. (1981) 'Visual results after removal of congenital cataracts before the age of 1 year.' *Canadian Journal of Ophthalmology*, **16**, 19–21.

Prendiville, A., Schulenberg, W.E. (1988) 'Clinical factors associated with retinopathy of prematurity.' *Archives of Disease in Childhood*, **63**, 522–527.

Ramatullah, L., Underwood, B., Thulsiraj, R.D., Milton, R.C., Ramaswarmy, K., Ramatullah, R., Babu, G. (1990) 'Reduced mortality among children in southern India receiving a small weekly dose of vitamin A.' *New England Journal of Medicine*, **323**, 929–935.

Rankin, S.J.A., Tubman, T.R.J., Halliday, H.L., Johnston, S.S. (1992) 'Retinopathy of prematurity in surfactant treated infants.' *British Journal of Ophthalmology*, **76**, 202–204.

Reddy, V., Rao, V., Arunjyothi, S., Reddy, M. (1989) 'Conjunctival impression cytology for assessment of vitamin A status.' *American Journal of Clinical Nutrition*, **50**, 814–817.

Riise, R., Flage, T., Hansen, E., Rosenberg, T., Rudanko, S-L., Viggosson, G., Warburg, M. (1992) 'Visual impairment in Nordic children. I: Nordic registers and prevalence data.' *Acta Ophthalmologica*, **70**, 145–154.

Rosenberg, T. (1987) 'Visual impairment in Danish children.' *Acta Ophthalmologica*, **65**, 110–117.

—— Flage, T., Hansen, E., Rudanko, S-L., Viggosson, G., Riise, R. (1992) 'Visual impairment in Nordic children. II: Aetiological factors.' *Acta Ophthalmologica*, **70**, 155–164.

Ross, C. (1992) 'Influence of vitamin A on the immune response.' *In:* West, K.P. (Rapporteur) *Bellagio Meeting on Vitamin A Deficiency and Childhood Mortality.* New York: Helen Keller International, pp. 28–31.

Royal National Institute for the Blind (1985) *Initial Demographic Study 1985. A Review of the Available Data on the Visually Disabled Population.* London: RNIB.

Sandford-Smith, J.H., Whittle, H.C. (1979) 'Corneal ulceration following measles in Nigerian children.'

British Journal of Ophthalmology, **63**, 720–724.

Schulenberg, W.E., Prendiville, A., Ohri, R. (1987) 'Natural history of retinopathy of prematurity.' *British Journal of Ophthalmology*, **71**, 837–843.

Seiberth, V., Linderkamp, O. (1989) 'Akute retinopathia praematurorum: Verlagerung des Manifestationsrisikos zu extrem unreifen Fruhgeborenen durch die neonatale Intensivmedizin.' *Fortschritte der Ophthalmologie*, **86**, 626–630.

Sheppard, R.W., Crawford, J.S. (1973) 'The treatment of congenital cataracts.' *Survey of Ophthalmology*, **17**, 340–347.

Shrivastva, S., Vajpayee, R.B., Sharma, Y.R. (1988) 'Vision in childhood aphakia.' *Indian Journal of Ophthalmology*, **36**, 123–125.

Singha, S.K., D'Souza, S.W., Rivlin, E., Chiswick, M.L. (1990) 'Ischaemic brain lesions diagnosed at birth in preterm infants: clinical events and developmental outcome.' *Archives of Disease in Childhood*, **65**, 1017–1020.

Sommer, A. (1982) *Field Guide to the Detection and Control of Xerophthalmia*. Geneva: WHO.

—— Tarwotjo, I., Djunaedi, E., West, K.P., Tilden, R.L., Loeden, A.A., Tilden, R., Mele, L., and the Aceh Study Group (1986) 'Impact of vitamin A supplementation on childhood mortality: a randomised controlled community trial.' *Lancet*, **1**, 1169–1173.

Stannard, K.P., Mushin, A.S., Gamsu, H.R. (1989) 'Screening for retinopathy of prematurity in a regional neonatal intensive care unit.' *Eye*, **3**, 371–378.

Stewart-Brown, S.L., Haslum, M.N. (1988) 'Partial sight and blindness in children of the 1970 birth cohort at 10 years of age.' *Journal of Epidemiology and Community Health*, **42**, 17–23.

Taylor, D. (1979) 'Amblyopia in bilateral infantile and juvenile cataract. Relationship to timing of treatment.' *Transactions of the Ophthalmological Society of the United Kingdom*, **99**, 170–175.

—— (1981) 'Choice of surgical technique in the management of congenital cataract.' *Transactions of the Ophthalmological Society of the United Kingdom*, **101**, 114–117.

—— (1982) 'Developments in the treatment of cataract. Treacher Collins Prize Essay.' *Transactions of the Ophthalmological Society of the United Kingdom*, **102**, 441–453.

—— (1985) 'Cataracts in childhood.' *Journal of the Royal Society of Medicine*, **78**, 1–3.

—— Rice, N.S.C. (1982) 'Congenital cataract, a cause of preventable child blindness.' *Archives of Disease in Childhood*, **57**, 165–167.

Tidjani, O., Grunitsky, B., Guérin, N., Lévy-Bruhl, D., Lecam, N., Xuereff, C., Tatagan, K. (1989) 'Serological effects of Edmonston-Zagreb, Schwartz, and AIK-C measles vaccine strains given at ages 4–5 or 8–10 months.' *Lancet*, **2**, 1357–1360.

Toyofuku, H., Hirose, T., Schepens, C.L. (1980) 'Retinal detachment following congenital cataract surgery. 1. Peroperative findings in 114 eyes.' *Archives of Ophthalmology*, **98**, 669–675.

Underwood, B.A. (1990a) 'Methods of assessment of vitamin A status.' *Journal of Nutrition*, **120**, 1459–1463.

—— (1990b) 'Vitamin A prophylaxis in developing countries: past experiences and future prospects.' *Nutrition Reviews*, **48**, 265–274.

Van der Pol, B.A.E. (1986) 'Causes of visual impairment in children.' *Documenta Ophthalmologica*, **61**, 223–228.

Veen, S., Ens-Dokkum, M.H., Schreuder, A.M., Verlooke-Vanhorick, S.P., Brand, R., Ruys, J.H. (1991) 'Impairments and handicaps of very preterm and very low birth weight infants at five years of age.' *Lancet*, **338**, 33–36.

Vijayaraghavan, K., Radhaiah, G., Prakasam, B.S., Sarma, K.V.R., Reddy, V. (1990) 'Effect of massive dose vitamin A on mortality in Indian children.' *Lancet*, **336**, 1342–1345.

West, K.P., Pokhrel, R.P., Katz, J., LeClerq, S.C., Kharty, S.K., Shrestha, S.R., Pradman, E.K., Tioelsch, J.M., Pandey, M.R., Sommer, A. (1991) 'Efficiency of vitamin A in reducing preschool child mortality in Nepal.' *Lancet*, **338**, 67–71.

Whittle, H.C., Campbell, H., Rahman, S., Armstrong, J.R.M. (1990) 'Antibody persistence in Gambian children after high-dose Edmonston-Zagreb measles vaccine.' *Lancet*, **336**, 1046–1048.

Wong, F. (1987) 'A new phase in the study of human inherited eye disease.' *Archives of Ophthalmology*, **105**, 1039–1041.

World Health Organization (1982) *Control of Vitamin A Deficiency and Xerophthalmia. Report of a Joint WHO/UNICEF/USAID/Helen Keller International/IVACG meeting. Technical Report Series 672*. Geneva: WHO.

—— (1986) *Conjunctivitis of the Newborn. Prevention and Treatment at the Primary Health Care Level.* Geneva: WHO.

—— (1991) 'Prevention of blindness—Prevalence and causes of blindness and low vision, Benin.' *Weekly Epidemiological Record*, **66**, 337–340.

—— (1992) *Prevention of Childhood Blindness.* Geneva: WHO.

INDEX

211